Praise for Mitch Stevens

As the publisher of *Uniquely You Magazine*, I have had the honor of sharing hundreds of stories from the special needs and disabled communities—stories of resilience, advocacy, joy, and everyday life that too often go unseen. I am also the mom of an autistic son, a role that has profoundly shaped how I view the world, language, and the systems that surround disability. *Transcending Labels* deeply resonated with me because it reflects what I've learned both personally and professionally: people are not defined by diagnoses, and connection begins when we are willing to truly see one another.

This book challenges us to pause and examine the labels we so easily use—sometimes for clarity, sometimes for convenience, but often without realizing the limitations they impose. Mitch invites readers to look beyond categories and instead lean into curiosity, empathy, and authentic relationship. As a parent, I know how often my son is seen through the lens of autism before he is seen as a child with humor, interests, struggles, and gifts. This book gives language and perspective to what so many families experience every day.

What makes *Transcending Labels* especially powerful is its emphasis on shared humanity. Disability is not a separate experience reserved for "others"—it is part of the human story. Through real-life narratives and thoughtful reflection, Mitch reminds us that connection is not about fixing or changing someone, but about honoring dignity, voice, and belonging. This is the kind of mindset shift our communities, schools, workplaces, and faith spaces desperately need.

I believe this book is not only timely, but necessary. It is a call to move from awareness to action, from assumptions to understanding, and from labels to lasting connection. For families like mine—and for anyone who desires a more inclusive and compassionate world—Transcending Labels offers both hope and a practical path forward.

~ Jamie Olson

TRANSCENDING LABELS

Conversations that Break Barriers and Build Understanding

MITCH STEVENS

KI Productions

Transcending Labels:
Conversations to Break Barriers and Build Understanding
Second Edition
Copyright © 2026 by Mitch Stevens

Paperback ISBN: 978-1-961605-66-4

KI Productions
Noblesville, IN

All Worldwide Rights Reserved.
All rights reserved. No part of this book may be reproduced, stored in a retrieval system or transmitted, in any form or by any means, electronic, mechanical, recorded, photocopied, or otherwise, without the prior written permission of the copyright owner, except by a reviewer who may quote brief passages in a review.

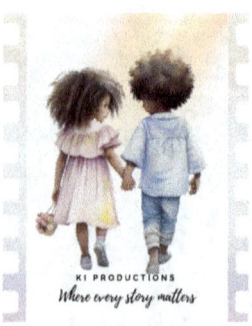

Contents

Foreword	vii
Preface	xi
Introduction	xiii
1. A Shot to Remember	1
2. The Wonderful Cindy Gajus	9
3. My Buddy, Steve	21
4. Challenges with Curriculum	37
5. Typical Students Getting Involved	43
6. Inclusion Beyond the Classroom	55
7. Disabled 365: Making a Difference in the Community	61
8. Siblings: Seeing Beyond the Disability with the Hunt Family	75
9. Siblings: Seeing Beyond Disability with Susan Conroy	93
10. Parents Seeing Beyond the Disability with Steve and Colleen Hunt	107
11. Advice for High School Students/Treating People the Right Way	127
12. Independent Living	139
13. Moments That Matter Most	147
14. From Rob's Perspective	155
15. The Power of Inclusion	161
BONUS: Blog	173
Acknowledgments	183
Resources	185

Foreword

I first met Mitch Stevens long before I ever imagined I would be writing a foreword for his book.

I knew of Mitch's father growing up through competing on the baseball diamond. Years later I watched Mitch as a young kid playing on the same team as my son James, on the football field. Mitch was one of the smallest players out there, but already someone who stood out. There was just something about him. You could see it even then. Fast forward more than a decade, and Mitch reentered our lives in a much more meaningful way when my youngest son, Rob, became the manager for his high school basketball team.

Rob has Down syndrome. He is capable, articulate, funny, deeply relational, and—like every person—far more than any label could ever describe. Mitch, who was a senior and a team captain at the time, didn't treat Rob like a project or a box to check. He treated him like a teammate. Like a brother. Mitch and another senior captain, Adam Boyer, took Rob under their wing, holding him accountable when needed, encouraging him when he struggled, and welcoming him fully into the life of the team.

Foreword

What made that season so powerful wasn't just inclusion—it was relationship. Mitch stayed present. Long after the season ended, long after graduation, long after it would have been easy to move on, he stayed connected. To this day, he still makes time to take Rob to lunch when he's in town, to sit with him, talk with him, and simply be with him. That matters more than I can adequately put into words.

What you will discover in Transcending Labels is that this posture—this way of being with people—is who Mitch is at his core. He doesn't approach the disability community from a distance or from a place of assumed expertise. He approaches it as a learner. As a listener. As someone willing to ask hard questions and sit with honest answers. His interview-based approach is not accidental; it reflects deep respect. Mitch understands that when we speak about the lives of others, we have a responsibility to listen first.

This book captures real life. It doesn't sanitize the challenges, and it doesn't reduce people to stereotypes. Mitch introduces readers to individuals and families across the intellectual and developmental disability community, reminding us that there is no single story, no single box, no one way to belong. Every person has their own interests, gifts, struggles, humor, and dreams—just like anyone else.

I have often said this book should be required reading in junior high and high school. Young people today are surrounded by distractions, but they are also capable of great compassion if we invite them to see what is possible. Transcending Labels opens minds. It challenges assumptions. It asks readers to slow down, engage, and consider the possibilities that emerge when we choose presence over fear and relationship over distance.

For families like ours, this kind of engagement has lasting impact. Rob's experience in high school—being known,

Foreword

expected, included, and challenged by his peers—shaped who he is today. He has worked full-time for the past 8+ years, at one of the largest national banks in the country, he has full benefits and contributes meaningfully to his community. That didn't happen by accident. It happened because people like Mitch saw him for who he is and chose to walk alongside him.

My hope is that this book does not stay on a shelf. I hope it sparks conversations, book clubs, classroom discussions, and community action. I hope it encourages readers to move beyond school-based inclusion and ask what belonging looks like in adulthood—where isolation too often takes hold. Most of all, I hope it helps people understand that when we invest in one another, everyone wins: individuals, families, and communities alike.

~ Steve Hunt

Preface

Some lessons in life need to be taught to us several times over before they sink in. You know, the ones that Mom and Dad preached endlessly, yet somehow they fell on deaf ears. Some lessons, however, hit you so hard that there is no avoiding it. They open your eyes to a completely new way of thinking, and you cannot imagine a world before you thought this way; it becomes a part of your identity. A complete paradigm shift. This was my experience getting to know the special needs community at my high school.

Need a reminder as to why you should be grateful for what you have? A better understanding of what it means to focus on your strengths versus limitations? Or maybe just a course entitled 'Happiness 101.' Either way, this group has you covered. I always considered myself an empathetic person with a heart for other people (thank you, Mom). Building friendships with people who have special needs showed me what that really means.

In my professional life, I have been fortunate to be surrounded by leaders who genuinely care about personal growth and showing up for the most important people in their lives.

Preface

Strategies I have learned in the personal growth department have made a massive impact on my life, just as my relationships with the special needs community have. Ergo, we have this book.

As I write this, I'm not quite sure that this will fit into any traditional genre. I'm fine with that. The pages to follow are a collection of what has been on my heart to share for years; the immeasurable value of connecting with these people. There just so happen to be hints of 'self-help' suggestions in there, too. A bit of it is from my perspective, but a large portion comes from conversations with some of the best human beings that I have ever met.

Use this as a guide for how to treat individuals with special needs and/or disabilities in your community. Take a suggestion from one of the application sections if you feel so inclined. Or, simply enjoy some heartwarming accounts of what it means to truly see beyond disabilities.

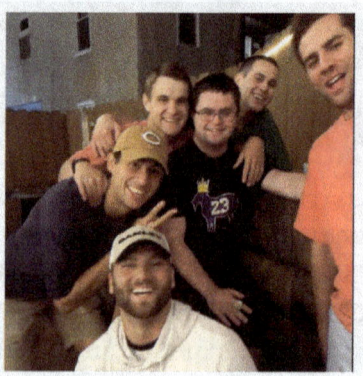

Robert's surprise 21st birthday celebration.

Introduction

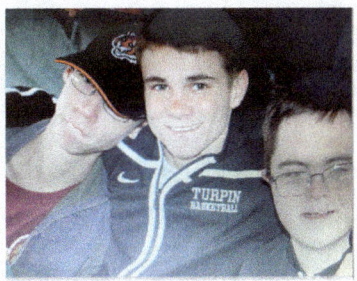

I was a special education major in college and spent two years in high school working alongside individuals with a variety of disabilities. To this day, I draw perspective from those experiences in many ways and it truly is a privilege whenever I get to spend time with these people. Anyone who has been connected to the special needs community can relate to that notion. I can attest to the fact that spending time with individuals with special needs and/or disabilities is always a worthwhile endeavor.

This book is a passion project of mine, and my hope is that it provides actionable information to all readers through way of

Introduction

reflection, brainstorming, and possibly discussion with others. I encourage you to take the time to pause and utilize those parts of the book. Learning to see beyond another person's differences or perceived disabilities in relationships, coaching, teaching, and everyday conversation is one of the most impactful lessons one can learn. Through personal stories and conversations with those closest to this wonderful community, I aim to show people why.

ONE

A Shot to Remember

"If you give people a chance, they shine."
Billy Connolly

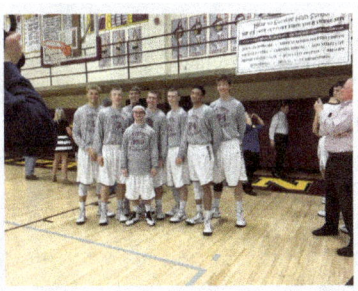

Robert and his Senior teammates pose ahead of his first appearance in a varsity game.

It was a Friday night in early February. The Turpin Spartans boys basketball team was taking on one of their biggest rivals, the Kings Knights. This was the final home game of the season, 'Senior Night.' Not to mention, both teams were competing for a better potential outlook in the state playoffs. But, Klinger Court was buzzing for reasons beyond that.

A four-year member of the varsity staff was going to get the opportunity to get into the game for the first time in his career, and everybody knew it. Former teammates came from all over, some making several-hour drives back to Cincinnati in order to see this moment.

In practice leading up to the game that week, the out of bounds play was rehearsed multiple times: 'hard jab at the right elbow, come off of the screen, put it up off the glass and in' — sounds simple, right? To put it only in those terms for Turpin senior Robert Hunt, however, would be a major disservice to the moment.

Being diagnosed with Down Syndrome at birth led to many challenges throughout his life. But now, after years of hard work, dedication, and always cheering on others in the spotlight, he finally had his opportunity—a chance to score a basket for his school in a varsity game.

"I think he wants to win more than anybody on our team," head coach Ryan Krohn said of Robert during the Fox19 Cincinnati feature of the moment. "He's here working hard, first one here all the time… he's just one of the guys."

Several of us former-Spartans sat together a couple rows behind the Turpin bench, nervously waiting for the call from Krohn to bring Rob into the game. I was anxious for this to happen, but I cannot fathom the emotions at play for his parents and siblings in attendance.

The coaches had agreed prior to the game that the play could happen in the first half, but none of us knew specifically when to expect it. This led to the longest quarter and a half of high school basketball you could possibly imagine; it felt like an eternity.

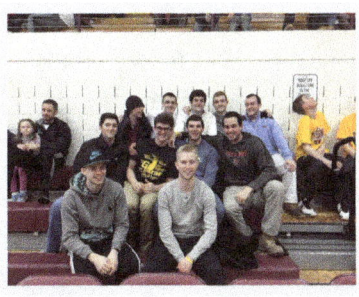

Turpin alumni there to cheer on Robert before the game.

Then finally, with only a few minutes remaining in the second quarter, it was time.

"Checking into the game for the Turpin Spartans, number 15, Rooobbbbeeeerrrrttt Huuuuuuunt!"

This is what I'd imagine the announcer said over the loudspeaker, but who am I kidding? Nothing was to be heard at that moment. The crowd was deafening. Rob got 'the point' from Coach Krohn, hopped up out of his seat, and bolted to the scorers table— from that point on, the energy in that gym was palpable.

Robert has a low-key, easy-going personality about him to put it mildly. He enjoys the spotlight as any of us do, but is generally a quiet and reserved guy. With that being said, even I was surprised at how calm and collected he was as he walked onto the court for the first time. It was as if he had it all rehearsed in his head for the past several years (I'd imagine that he did).

"Cool as the other side of the pillow," his father Steve would later say during the Fox19 special.

The head official was fully-prepared to meet him with a handshake and maybe even offer a word of encouragement before he headed onto the court. Rob had a different mentality. No joking around, no funny business. He gave the ref an emphatic high-five, followed by a dead-eyed glare straight into the sold-out student section as he waved his arms in the 'pump up the crowd' motion several times.

Seconds later, it was happening. Robert set up at the right elbow as his teammate was ready to inbound the ball. A few good friends and I stood across the court behind the Spartan bench, anxiety through the roof. We were nervous, Rob was not. A quick jab step, cut to the basket, and his shot is GOOD off of the glass! Pandemonium ensued at Klinger Court.

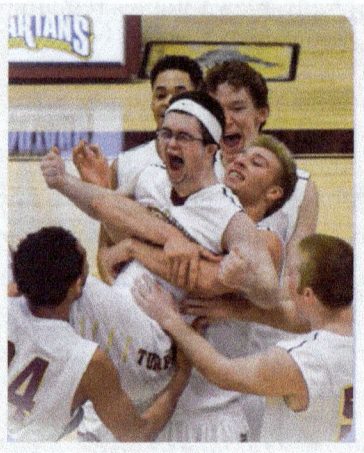

Robert's celebration with several teammates following the big shot.

> *I had so much fun. It was really awesome that I got to play and see how many people felt that emotion."*

To this day, that is the loudest roar I have heard from a crowd at Turpin. The competition and win-at-all-costs mentality involved in sports are certainly special. But, what happened that night for Robert in front of his closest friends and family transcended the 'W' or 'L' column. It was a truly human experience. Both sides could separate themselves from the game and turn their attention to what mattered most, which was including someone that truly deserved it.

Rob spent a majority of his childhood rooting on his older brothers, and then ultimately his teammates at Turpin. He was always excited to see people that he loved succeed. Is there a good chance that he spent lots of time fantasizing about playing, or wishing things were different so that he could be the star of the show? I'm sure, because who wouldn't think that way?

From personal experience, though, I cannot think of one time in my playing career in which Rob ever brought up that type of thing. He was pumped for us when we won, devastated when we lost, and that was it. He loved each of us, and that is the type of compassion and character shared by so many with special needs. This is also the number one reason why he was the heart and soul of Turpin basketball during those four years.

That was a powerful moment. For those who know the family, it was even sweeter. Many of you reading this may have experienced something similar or seen a story like this one on television. Being an avid sports fan, I see a few of them every year. For someone like Robert, though, what happens next? The moments of spotlight lit him and his family up in ways they'd never imagined when learning that their child would be born with Down Syndrome, but life goes on. I don't mean to take anything away from what happened that night because it was thrilling to see. We do not want to lose signature moments such as the one described above. The question I aim to tackle with this book, however, is 'how do we see beyond the perceived limitations of those with special needs in our day to day lives?'

Throughout this book, you'll read stories and insights from individuals with direct experience in this area. We will get back to Robert's story and conversations I had with a few of his family members, but first, I'd like to introduce you to Mrs. Cindy Gajus. Working with hundreds of students with special needs over her career, Cindy developed and honed the skills necessary to facilitate growth in each of them. She embodied seeing beyond the disabilities in others every day of teaching career.

REFLECTION

When reading about Robert's special moment, which emotions came up for you?

No matter how big or small, who can you create a special moment for in your life?

_____
_____
_____
_____
_____
_____
_____
_____
_____
_____

TWO

The Wonderful Cindy Gajus

"Working with those guys has been such a privilege, and I learned more from them than they could have ever learned from me. I'm not amazing because I help them– they're the amazing ones."
Cindy Gajus

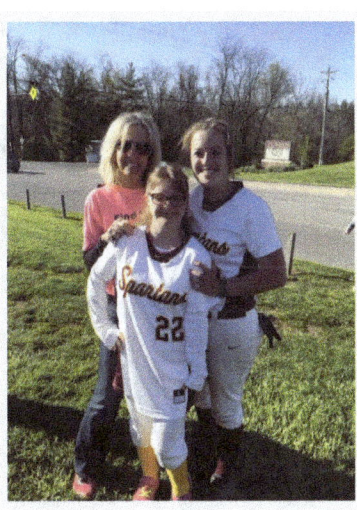

Cindy Gajus (left), poses with a student-aide and her student, Anne.

Our first introduction was during my junior year at Turpin High School. I was approached by one of my best friends, Alex Williams, about an after-school club that he and his sister had been attending. The club was called "Chillin' Chums," and was organized by Cindy. They met twice a month after school, and organized one fun outing each month as well. When I think about a deeper purpose for wanting to help and include individuals with special needs, I often think back to my time associated with Chillin' Chums.

Cindy's leadership of this group was inspiring to me in many ways. Now retired from teaching, she was kind enough to sit down with me to recount her impactful career in teaching. She is an expert in seeing beyond disabilities, whether it be in the classroom or post-education lifestyle.

Her first experience with inclusion was with a preschool classroom. She spent five years with these students. Approximately half of the students had disabilities, and half were typically-developing.

 It was so natural," she recalled. "All of the kids played and participated with each other, and fed off of each other. So, I'm thinking 'okay…why doesn't that go on as the kids get older?'"

To an extent, it makes sense to think that it would be more natural for students to embrace each other no matter their differences at a young age. It is also understandable that the disparity between typical students and those with special needs causes some issues in terms of classroom dynamics in the early-teen to teenager phase. Cindy saw what was working at the preschool and felt that she could recreate the connection regardless of the students' ages.

Fast-forward to chapter two of her career, she was leading the charge and making it happen with her students at Nagel Middle School. The "Chillin Chums" club initially started around this time. Cindy spent five years in a 'cross-categorical model' at Nagel, which consisted of about a dozen children with an extremely wide range of disabilities. She had students that would be considered cognitively low-functioning, as well as students with a few emotional disorders.

Her depiction of this classroom's dynamics are as follows, and I wish I could do justice with written words to the passion behind it.

"It was not an easy task. But every day, I had the support of a group of teachers at Nagel and a principal that was amazing," she started, as we both tried to stop ourselves from getting emotional.

She talked about learning where each student is emotionally, mentally, physically, and then tailoring instruction from there. However, when it's a group with wide-ranging abilities and disabilities, that can be a major challenge. Having a great team and in-depth preparation is the combination that led to success in Cindy's classroom.

> "It was a collective effort," she said. "Every week when we were discussing what we were going to be teaching, I would have my own plan for each student. So for each subject, we made adjustments depending on the student. If this person is in a wheelchair and the other students are going to be going around doing an experiment, what could we do? And that's where I could always come up with an intervention, some sort of gadget, or at least some purpose that person could have to be a part of the group and have a great experience."

I think this concept can certainly apply outside of the classroom for friends or parents of these individuals, too. Assessing what a fun event or get together is going to look like, and then making modifications to ensure that nobody is being left out or unable to enjoy the experience with everyone else.

> "Every day I went into the classroom, and the teachers were working with me, the other students were working with me, and they all made each other feel actively involved in the classroom. Everybody had high expectations. Everybody was working to their potential and learning together. Nobody was feeling sorry for anybody. All of the students expected each other to do the best that they could, and that happened day in, and day out at Nagel," she said.

This is a powerful example of people working together to make this beautiful concept of inclusion come to fruition at a high level. Notice that she made it a point to say that "nobody was feeling sorry for anybody." That is simply another way of saying that all team members were able to see beyond the disabilities and focus on the task at hand.

When it comes to individuals with disabilities, it can be easy and even natural for one to default to that mindset of feeling bad for them. We'll dive into this concept deeper in a moment, but approaching these individuals with the opposite mentality is much more beneficial for everybody involved. Those five years were a great opportunity for Cindy to prove to herself that successful inclusion could be executed with older students. As impactful as that stage of her career was, a few years into it she was offered her next opportunity, this time with Turpin High School.

"My boss told me that there was a group of parents that love inclusion, but they understand that their kids need more than that as they're getting older," she said, referring to parents of high school students at the time. "They want (their student) to learn skills so that they can live on their own someday and take care of themselves."

This was the beginning of what became the Life Skills program that defined the next couple decades of Cindy's career. It was centered around the need for understanding and development of real-world skills and concepts for individuals with special needs. The objective was not to eliminate or ignore traditional content taught during school. Instead, the purpose was to make an emphasis on looking for as many real-life experiences for her students, many of which they would not have encountered pre-graduation otherwise.

Many of the things they taught were out in the community, going to all of the familiar spots in the area. She wanted people in the community to get to know these students. There were specific times she recalled when they took the students grocery shopping to teach them how to do it on their own. Workers at Kroger would notice that one of her students was in an aisle alone, looking confused. The worker would let Cindy know that the student was out of place, but Cindy would reassure them that her and her staff knew exactly where that student was, but they wanted them to work through where to go next; she wanted it to be a growth opportunity.

"I was able to start that program at Turpin and it was supposed to be community-based. In my brain I was thinking, 'It's not just about school; it's about where we live, how we get places, how we live, our neighbors, etc. I really took it as a community effort to help my students," she said.

Cindy developed her own curriculum for this new program all in one summer prior to beginning at the high school. Her daughter helped her in this endeavor, providing her with materials and ideas for how to structure it with such a short window of time before day one. After her arrival at Turpin and the start of her new class, the next step was to figure out how to get other students involved.

Sure enough, as was the case for Cindy at Nagel Middle School, she was met with teachers at Turpin that were accepting, open, and willing to help. She was assisted by an amazing speech and language pathologist, Verna Donovan, and an exceptional pair of professionals on her team. Verna was in charge of many of their social skills classes. In addition, she would lead role-play sessions for the students leading up to events outside of the classroom. Cindy noted that Verna's leadership in this area was critical to students feeling comfortable and confident doing things such as going to school dances, sporting events, etc.

Another person who was integral to the program's success was science teacher Mrs. Corey Mullins. She was at the forefront of facilitating inclusion in the early years of the Life Skills program. Cindy approached her early on looking for an opportunity to collaborate.

> "I told her 'I've got so many students that love science, and I could teach them science but I'm not a science teacher. I would really love it if we could do something together'."

Of course, Mullins was more than willing to help. This process began with her providing Cindy's class with materials to facilitate science lessons and experiments. It then eventually evolved into something special when Mullins came to Cindy with ideas surrounding inclusion with the two classrooms.

> "'Your kids can teach my students something, and maybe we can teach you guys something!' So, my kids taught her students about their disabilities, and then her students did experiments with my students. It was within the core curriculum, but they were using microscopes, all of these materials that I didn't have, going on hikes—we spent the night at the zoo together, we did so many amazing things," Cindy recalled.

I found this early story of the program to be inspiring and a wonderful example of what can happen when a couple of passionate individuals decide to collaborate and take action on something that they wanted to bring to life. Sure, state standards and regulations (which we will refer to again) can sometimes put a bit of a stranglehold on teachers in this sense. However, this example of two individuals being determined to make it happen is powerful, and they did so while adhering to core curriculum guidelines, too! This experience inspired Cindy to connect with professors at the University of Cincinnati to do something similar. She shared with these teachers that her students were learning about their disabilities, how to advocate for themselves, and that it was going extremely well.

> "Before you knew it, my students were going to the University of Cincinnati and teaching students about their disabilities. I'm sitting in the front row watching them do this after practicing and practicing, and just watching them up there giving a speech about their

disabilities, I'm tearing up. I'm thinking that I wouldn't have the guts to do that, yet I'm having them do it?! But the rewards were so great."

I'm not crying, you're crying. Can you remember the first time you had to get up in front of a group and present to the class by yourself? Terrifying to most. For some, it elicits more fear than the thought of death itself, yet Cindy's students were up there doing it for students that were older than them!

Putting students in these types of scenarios was commonplace throughout her career. She developed a culture centered around growth and treating them as adults from an early stage. This is one of the key concepts I learned from working directly with Cindy: holding high expectations for all students. I found this to be particularly difficult in my early experiences working with students with special needs, and I think it is a valuable take on mindset for anyone who wants to support the empowerment of these individuals. She was determined to push these students (and, in many cases, the families of the students) out of their comfort zones. As a result, it helped everyone grow and get continually closer to being able to take care of themselves when they were no longer in the classroom. This is a mentality that Cindy brought every single day with each of her students, keeping a strong focus on preparing each individual person for life after school. She constantly looked for areas of opportunity, particularly those that may make things difficult for people with special needs in the 'real world.'

The program was such a success that it resulted in Cindy receiving the Franklin Walter Outstanding Educator Award from the state of Ohio in 2002. She then got the opportunity to go to an event in Columbus to speak on how they were able to make it all happen.

There are certain undeniable limitations associated with the students in Cindy's classroom. The idea of pushing those limits, then, is not to say that we should ignore the inherent struggles that any of these individuals experience; it is the concept of challenging ourselves to look at it from the opposite perspective as much as possible. To see beyond the disabilities.

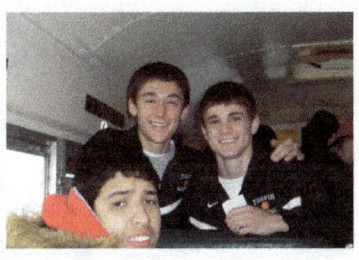

Alex Williams (left), with Mitch and one of Cindy's students, Mauricio.

One of the most important developments in her Life Skills program was the growth of the aforementioned Chillin' Chums Club at Turpin. This group was designed for all students, not only those with disabilities, to come together for arts and crafts projects, fun group games, and ultimately field trips out in the 'real world.'

When Alex first encouraged me to attend, not all that different from trying anything new, I was a bit nervous to go the first time. I knew that many of the students that would attend, help facilitate activities, and lead the way had been 'regulars' for quite some time. They had already built relationships with each other and created a true sense of community prior to my joining. I was also apprehensive because I had minimal experience interacting with anyone with special needs; I was worried that I might not be able to understand or connect with them. Boy, was I wrong. I've always considered myself to be fairly outgoing and apt at speaking with others, but the instant connections had nothing to do with me. I quickly learned that a majority of individuals in the class were extremely outgoing themselves, and they welcomed me with open arms.

This is a concept I'd like to expand upon for just a minute; first, the idea of being nervous or unsure of how to approach building relationships in these scenarios. I would imagine this is common for a typically-functioning person.

'What would I talk about with that person? What if I say something that could offend a parent, guardian, or friend of that individual? How do I approach this individual with empathy for their current situation, but not treating them and their loved ones as if I feel sorry for them?'

These were some of the thoughts that went through my mind as I joined Chillin' Chums and carefully tried to navigate conversations with the members of the group, as well as the student-helpers. These same questions guide my behavior toward individuals with special needs and disabilities to this day. I am here to tell anyone reading this that those thoughts are 100% normal to have, but they shouldn't get in the way of what could become some of your most cherished friendships. The students in that group showed me immediately that they were easy-going, happy, and so excited to have me there, all before truly getting to know me. Sounds like an elementary concept that we could all learn to embody a little more in our lives in general, right?

I am forever grateful to Alex for encouraging me to show up to that first meeting because it has altered my perspective on life in the most positive of ways. Most of us automatically make judgments about another person when we first meet, and I don't think that is avoidable—it's almost automatic in our brains. I do, however, think that all of us can work on our ability to quickly move past our preconceived notions and adopt an open mind regardless of who it is that we meet. I am, by no means, perfect in this area, but being a part of this group resulted in dramatic improvements. Not to mention, without this group I would never have connected with one of my favorite human beings of all-time: Stephen Cornell.

REFLECTION

In your next interaction with someone with special needs or a disability, consider asking yourself: "How much of a focus am I putting on their capabilities instead of the perceived limitations?

How much of our conversations and activities together, no matter how small they may seem, are focused on the growth of this person?"

THREE

My Buddy, Steve

"When we raise the bar, people rise to meet it."
Colleen Patrick-Goudreau

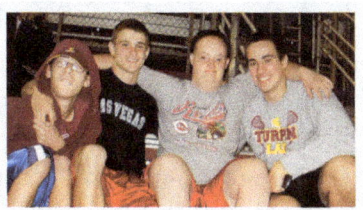

Stephen Cornell (left), Mitch, Devin Pable, and another basketball teammate, Adam Boyer (right), taking in a Turpin soccer game.

I SHARED with Cindy that my natural inclination when first being introduced to the group was to sort of 'baby' them. I found myself tempted to allow certain behaviors to go unaddressed, even if they were not things that a typical high school student should be doing. In my opinion, this is such a prevalent matter whether it is a teacher, a parent, or someone like myself working with these individuals in a student aide capacity. It is most people's natural mindset to lower their expectations immediately. 'Oh, this student is not supposed to know how to behave in this certain setting. We'll let that one slide,' one might think. Cindy begs to differ, and this quality in her as an educator made all the difference in the growth of her students. This applies no matter how basic the behavior may seem.

One of the seemingly simple tasks that was important for Stephen to master was crossing the street. Obviously, this was crucial to his parents in order for them to feel that he can be safe on his own. Security guards at Turpin and Verna Donovan would drive around the school's campus and teach Stephen how to do just that.

"He took it so seriously," Cindy commented. "It was adorable to watch, and it was an important lesson for him." She also added that Turpin's principal, Peggy Johnson, was instrumental in giving her free reign to do so many of these things during a school day.

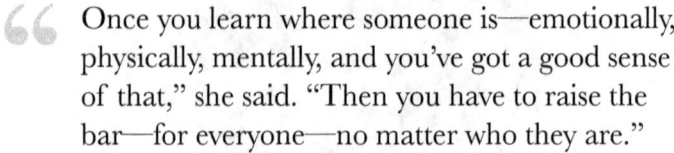

> Once you learn where someone is—emotionally, physically, mentally, and you've got a good sense of that," she said. "Then you have to raise the bar—for everyone—no matter who they are."

It took time for me to learn 'where Stephen was' when working with him in the group and one-on-one. Thankfully, I was fortunate to learn from the best with Cindy running the show. Steve deals with severe cognitive impairments that make it exceptionally difficult to retain information, communicate with others, and perform some of life's tasks that many don't even think about on a day-to-day basis. Despite the clear challenges at hand, his positive energy and enthusiasm for life are infectious. For whatever reason, he took a particular interest in me within minutes of my first time hanging out with the group. I cannot tell you what we did in the classroom that afternoon, nor can I recall any words that were exchanged between the two of us. I can, however, vividly illustrate the feeling I had leaving that day.

> *"I've learned that people will forget what you said, people will forget what you did, but people will never forget how you made them feel."*
> Maya Angelou

This is one of my favorite quotes in general, specifically because it sums up the impact it can have when one chooses inclusion and to connect with the special needs community. I left Turpin High School that day feeling like a million bucks, and I had Steve to thank for it. If I were able to wave a magic wand and take away 99% of his daily struggles, they would still far outweigh anything I have to bear. Yet, during our time together, I wasn't worried about a test coming up, the girl I liked in school, a buddy of mine that didn't want to hang out last weekend— none of it. And the more I spent time with him and that group, the more accustomed I became to not worrying about those things at all. Sure, everyone has their own demons and anxieties to deal with on a daily basis, and those have never fully gone away for me, either. Those are a necessary part of life. But, being introduced to this community put a huge dent in that. I found it nearly impossible to be around Stephen and simultaneously feeling upset or angry.

Because it was such a positive experience the first time I went, I began to make the meetings a more consistent activity. By the time the next school year rolled around, it was a full-blown part of my identity. It still is to this day, and there are few things in life that could make me more proud.

Another component of my experience were the numerous opportunities that Cindy facilitated for students outside of the classroom. It started with her effort to bring a group to a Friday night football game. This was a bold proposition, particularly to the families involved. If you have little experience with individuals with disabilities, I'd encourage you to put yourself into the shoes of a parent for this section. Worrying about something as small as attending the school's sporting event could sound like overkill at first, but there are so many factors at play. The desire of a parent to make sure their son or daughter is treated well, not taken advantage of, and embraced by their peers cannot be overstated. This is precisely where a committed and passionate leader like Cindy came into play for the Turpin parents, easing those anxieties every step of the way.

She added to this thought specifically as it relates to Stephen.

"Take (Stephen) for example… Once I realized his capabilities, now I'm going to raise the bar for him. I'm going to probably try to bring the parents along, too, because I did a lot of scary things."

To say that some of the things she tried with students were "scary" is not at all an exaggeration. During our conversation, she specifically recounted that first experience at the football game.

"I remember the first time I told some parents I wanted the kids to go to a football game and they were scared to death. When we got there, I just started to go back farther and farther in the stands and watch everybody interact with one another. It was amazing to see other students saying to my kids, 'hey come down here and sit with us and cheer!' To me, that was the other students essentially saying 'come and be a part of our team.' That inclusiveness allowed my students to feel like 'oh wow, this is my school, and I'm doing what everybody else does!'"

I mentioned Mrs. Verna Donovan's role earlier, and according to Cindy, she was pivotal to making these events run smoothly. For weeks leading up to the game, they practiced every part of their experience numerous times. They role-played walking up the hill to the field, holding onto the railings in the stands, seeing where to go to be a part of the student section—all of it. The ultimate goal was to ensure that the students were comfortable and confident going into these new experiences.

When it came to school dances, they would practice how to dance, how to be appropriate in that setting, as well as covering rules for being respectful of others in that environment. For field trips, such as the one I will detail later to Cincinnati's Kenwood Mall, there were months of preparation leading up to it. The students were responsible for earning money on their own for nearly two months before going to the mall. This could be as simple as doing chores around their house, or doing something to help their neighbors out.

"We wanted to instill the concept of thinking outside of themselves," Cindy said. "The idea was to teach our kids the process of earning their own money to be able to buy Christmas presents for their friends and family. We made a list of who to buy for, practiced how to give the proper amount of money for an item to a cashier, etc."

She went on to add that it became such a source of pride for her students to do these things on their own. That right there is the definition of inclusion to me. Sure, when most people think of inclusion, they jump to the classroom setting and the idea of giving students with disabilities an equal opportunity to learn with their peers. While that is certainly a key component of inclusion, it is only that— one component. Being confident and comfortable within their communities is a separate and equally important part of it. When you add the fact that typically-functioning high school students were a part of most of these experiences, putting others with special needs before themselves in those social settings, it had such a lasting impact on those kids and their families.

I recall being told a story during my elementary years about a boy who was in sixth grade at my school (I was in fourth). He chose to sit with a fellow classmate with special needs because the student was about to eat lunch by himself. He was recognized in front of the whole school for his kindness and *bravery*, being the one person to put himself out there and join his classmate. I can still remember the guy's first and last name, and the way I felt hearing that story, and it was 20 years ago as I write this. Every little act of kindness towards this community matters.

When I think back fondly on my high school experience, so many of the positives can be attributed to the true sense of community, belongingness, and being a part of something bigger than myself. These feelings were mostly associated with sports. If we can take that concept and make it a primary focus to make all students, not only those with special needs or disabilities, feel like they are an important part of the group—then we've really got something. This sense of unity is created mostly during the times outside of the classroom when students get the opportunity to be social and connect with one another. Cindy went on to describe in more detail how impactful experiences like those were for her and her students.

"These moments still make me so emotional because there were so many times of connectedness that is so natural, and some people don't realize and still haven't experienced such beauty," she said.

A central theme throughout my conversation with Cindy was a genuine desire to create as many of these moments for her students as possible. It all started with a belief that they would thrive in these scenarios in the same manner that a typical student would. Many of the best leaders, managers, and coaches are often described by their mentees as being someone who 'believed in them before they truly believed in themselves.' It is no different for a teacher, of course, and Cindy embodied this characteristic as well as any leader I know.

"Believing in Stephen, making him feel like and know that he is an important person who is capable was huge. It started with earning the parents' trust. So, it was first my job to know the student's potential. And then, it was to respect the parents, but also try to bring them along, too," she said.

The biggest area of opportunity for our society, in her opinion, is helping to change the mindset of the people that work with these individuals after they are out of the classroom. She highlighted the importance of this being a community effort in our day to day lives, not just every now and then at a football game or public event. Cindy is especially passionate about the idea of a couple former students getting the opportunity to live together on their own. Once again, it all comes back to the growth, confidence, and increased self-worth and dignity of these individuals. A few of her past students recently made this move into their own house and they are thriving in their new situation. The families of these gentlemen made the decision to pair them together based on knowledge of each individual's strengths and weaknesses to ensure that it would be a good fit for everyone involved.

"Those four guys recently moved into a Smart Home, and this house is so tech-y that you couldn't burn it down if you wanted to. You couldn't even scald yourself in the shower, and it has every safety feature you could imagine, so that over time they won't need anyone to come and check on them," she said. "Right now, they are down to someone coming to check on them about four hours a day."

This is a major step in the right direction, and I was pleased to hear that my hometown community is making this a focus. A key issue with these living situations currently, Cindy feels, is that the Direct Support Professionals (DSPs) charged with helping these individuals are not necessarily operating from that high-expectations mentality we referenced earlier. A DSP's job is to work closely with people of all ages who have intellectual and developmental disabilities, but their biggest responsibilities occur when traditional schooling has ended. Cindy made it clear that she has great respect for DSPs and the role they play in these people's lives, but feels adjustments need to be made to the overall approach of some.

"Many of the (DSPs) want only to help (people with special needs), instead of believing in them and having expectations of them," she said. "So, the mindset of care-taking versus having expectations of them. If we could change the mindset of DSPs and pay them what they deserve, we could save a lot of money and make big improvements to the current system. 24-hour care is not necessary for (the four guys in the Smart Home). And more importantly, what does it do to their dignity? You learn all these skills, you get all this motivation to move out, and then somebody comes in and treats you like you're younger than you are," she added.

Cindy expanded upon this idea of not needing 24-hour care by pointing out that it can save state governments a lot of money and make the systems for independent living more efficient. If DSPs are trained to find out the abilities of the people under their care first, they can cut down on hours of supervision.

"This will also help with how they house people with special needs together," she said. "Maybe you have one person with strong mental abilities, but they are older and in a wheelchair. If you pair that person with an individual who struggles cognitively, they could help each other out. This is just an example, but thinking more creatively about it is what matters."

This type of creative thinking could help families such as the Hunts and Conroys (which we'll get to later) to feel like they have better options for their son. Cindy wants this conversation to continue, particularly because of the unfortunate reality that most parents of people with special needs are going to pass away before their child. Circumstances are different for each family, but having a safe plan in place is crucial.

TAKEAWAYS ON INDEPENDENT LIVING

1. Independent Living is not currently the best option for all individuals with special needs and their families.

2. We have a great deal of respect for anyone who decides to make their career based around positively influencing this community.

3. If a family's goal for their son or daughter is to live independently, the system needs to be set up to empower that individual. 24-hour monitoring, while well-intentioned, does the opposite.

The accessibility of these homes based on family financial standing is another area of concern. We will address this in my conversation with Steve and Colleen Hunt.

Another component of inclusion outside of the classroom has to do with specific communities supporting these individuals in a more respectful manner. For Cindy, this ranges from the people that may live on the same street and see them on a daily basis to practicing a simple common courtesy in a public setting such as a grocery store.

"If our community can be more accepting of people with special needs living in their neighborhoods, to understand that they are not scary people, that would make a huge difference," she said. "The Smart House right now? I think all of the neighbors understand that those guys are pretty cool people. And it's not even as much about being scared; it's more of a lack of knowledge. If you see somebody struggling, strike up a conversation with them at the very least."

In over 20 years working alongside people with special needs and/or disabilities, Cindy witnessed numerous interactions between her students and the general public. At times, these interactions were constructive, and at times they were not. I asked her to share advice on how to approach encounters like these, particularly for those who lack experience with people in this community.

"Be a little more patient, give them more time to order their food, to pay for their groceries, etc. And do not give them money for their food, because I saw that happen a lot, people wanting to pay for them when that was a learning opportunity. The community needs to continue to support in a way that is respectful and with higher expectations."

The first opportunity that I had to see these students in a public setting came during my junior year at Turpin. About six months after being introduced to the group, I was invited to join the field trip to Kenwood Mall in Cincinnati. It was a Friday morning in early December, coincidentally the day of our team's first regular season basketball game. We all piled into the bus in anticipation of the big day at the mall. This was the first field trip I had experienced since grade school, and I was PUMPED. I've never really cared for going to the mall, but an opportunity to spend the day hanging out with this group instead of traditional classes? Yes, please.

I was primarily responsible for assisting Stephen, which is a lot of fun, but definitely comes with its challenges as well. It was extremely easy for him to get distracted and start lagging behind the group, or to become locked into something exciting he saw in the mall (it was Christmas time, after all). If we were hanging out on our own time, this would not have been a problem at all. We could spend half of the time checking out the decorations surrounding Santa (we'll come back to that), and half of the time in the food court. However, given that we were on a specific schedule with the Life Skills group, it required that I come up with some creative ideas to get him moving.

"Steve, c'mon, it's a race!!" I said, about ten separate times as I would start jogging ahead of him. He would begin his old familiar (and adorable) laugh and start slowly running towards myself and the rest of the group.

"Steve, what's Devin doing?!" This one was particularly effective because Devin is a great friend of his, so realizing that he was behind the group and Devin was not? Definitely some effective motivation. Anyway, it was a constant effort throughout the day to keep my guy moving. On top of that, winter is a heavy allergy season for him. This meant lots of helping him use his handkerchief if he was having issues in that department. At certain moments, that led to our trip becoming a little bit messy because this was not a thing (at least at the time) that he was able to take care of on his own, and needed to be addressed immediately when it happened.

When it comes to these difficulties, I have a couple of thoughts and reasons for putting them in here. None of them are to complain, so, I hope it didn't come across that way. First of all, I do think it is an aspect worth noting for anyone considering going on this type of career path, or getting more involved with these students if you're currently in school. At risk of stating the obvious here, there are challenges. While I absolutely love these guys, it is not the easiest thing in the world to care for them, even if just for a day or one class period per day. Secondly, helping someone with special needs through these types of things is what makes the experience rewarding and even more of a reason to get involved.

> *You become someone that they can rely on, that they will look to for a helping hand, and that feeling is incredible.*

During my meeting with Cindy, she also recalled this outing to Kenwood Mall (how could any of us forget). However, she reminded me of a part of that day that somehow had completely slipped my mind, and perfectly encapsulates the lengths she was willing to go to in the interest of helping her kids.

Given that the group visited in December, as soon as we walked in we saw Santa sitting there. Stephen got extremely excited and wanted to sit on Santa's lap. Still being relatively new to the whole 'raise the bar' concept that guided Cindy's teaching, I thought nothing of it initially. For her, on the other hand, it was a massive learning opportunity.

"So right there at Kenwood Mall," she said, "I called his Mom and said 'I want you to know that this is what I saw… would you be comfortable with me talking to Stephen about the fact that there is no Santa Claus or is this something that you think you could take up?'"

Talk about a difficult conversation to have! These are the ones, though, that make the biggest impact especially on young people. Cindy did not downplay the challenging nature of bringing this up to a parent.

"I'm a parent and a grandparent, so I understand both perspectives. For me, it's always been: how is (Stephen) going to be the best person he can be, be respected, and have dignity? And if someone sees him in public doing something like this, or if he's out working a job and talking about Santa Claus, he becomes someone who can easily be taken advantage of," she added.

Powerful ideas for any teacher, parent, grandparent, or anyone else working with these communities:

***Mitch, these aren't ideas, they are questions. Let's use them as Reflection Questions

1. **How am I helping this individual become the best person that they can be?**
2. **How am I helping them to feel and become more respected by others?**
3. **Do they have a sense of dignity, and I am helping to facilitate the growth in that area?**

She went on to note that Stephen's mother decided to have the conversation with him on her own. The overarching point Cindy made on this subject is that even though it was difficult, it ended up being just fine. Sure, Stephen was a little mentally rattled from learning that there is no Santa Claus. But, again at risk of stating the obvious, there is so much joy surrounding Christmas that doesn't have anything to do with Santa or presents. It was crucial that he moved on from believing otherwise. Cindy understands the gravity of these types of situations for parents, but also that the result of a more mature individual in their child is so much better.

The trip wound up being a huge success from my perspective in multiple ways. First, this was the most responsibility I had been given to care for an individual with disabilities. I learned a lot about what it takes to be of assistance outside of the school for much longer than a 50-minute class period. In addition, I was reminded even more of the infectious attitudes on display in these students. I mentioned that we had our first basketball game of the season later that day, and sports are something that I have always taken seriously. Not to mention, this was the first time I would have the opportunity to play on the varsity level. To say I was anxious for that night would be a gross understatement. The entire week leading up to it, I did everything I could to keep my mind off of the game. Nothing really worked until this trip. I found that spending this quality time with people who are genuinely happy and grateful despite their challenges forced me to be present with them throughout. I cannot say that I didn't think about the game at all while we were at the mall. After all, two of my teammates were on the trip and we all wore our game day warmup jackets, for goodness sake. But, those thoughts were few and far between, and the Life Skills group instilled in me that ability to be present; that is a powerful gift.

On the note of facilitating maturity in her students, a situation similar to the Santa issue occurred when Cindy took the kids for an overnight summer camping trip. A young girl named Anne joined the group as an incoming freshman, so this was her first experience with the group. That first day, she showed up with her 'Wooby,' AKA a 'blanky' that she still carried with her almost all of the time. She had a strong emotional attachment to this blanket, which any parent can understand. I believe 'Woody' from Toy Story was my must-have back in the day. But, of course, that was when I was five years old.

Cindy's mentality around expectations and a student's dignity showed up right away, and a similar conversation occurred with the girl's mother. She would offer to have the tough conversation for the parent, but always made sure she did not overstep her boundaries by giving the parent the opportunity to do it instead.

"After that conversation, her mother still tells me to this day 'I can't believe that it was that simple for me to show it to her, box it up, put it away and that it was going to be okay. And I allowed her to do that.' And I got respect from her parents right away after that because she didn't need that blanket, it looked ridiculous at her age."

Although it is obvious that it doesn't make much sense for a high school student to be carrying something like this around, again I'd like to point out that it is not easy to put the proverbial foot down on things like that for a student with special needs. Cindy did, though, time and time again, because she knew that even something that small could set a positive precedent for growth in maturity. Fast-forward only a couple of years? As of writing this, Anne has been in two weddings, she's working at Kroger, and has been living on her own with three roommates for two months now. In addition, she earned herself a pay raise after five years working at Kroger. All of these accomplishments bring Cindy so much pride, and she added that it was amazing to have recently been invited to Anne's first housewarming party.

"It's so heartwarming to see how happy these guys are now that they've moved out of the house just like their siblings," she said. "But, if we would have kept on with that whole mindset of 'she's got a disability, she still believes in Santa Claus, she's allowed to have a blanky,' that wouldn't be the case. So, along the way you're raising expectations of both the parents and the student, but how rewarding?"

REFLECTION

Who are the people in your life that lift you up? Who is somebody that consistently makes you feel good when you're with them?

Who or what in your life causes you to lock in and be fully present with what you are doing?

How might you make an effort to spend more time with those people and/or doing those things?

_____

_____

_____

_____

_____

_____

_____

_____

_____

_____

FOUR

Challenges with Curriculum

"There are so many resources out there now, but you can feel good about talking to your intervention specialist. They became a teacher out of their passion and wanting to make a difference."
Cindy Gajus

CINDY's impactful career lasted a whopping 20 years before she finally decided to retire from teaching in 2016. With clearly so much passion still left for the field, I asked her to give some feedback on why she made the decision to move on, and specifically what she would change about the current school system.

It was starting to be too focused on academics and losing life skills, and it was getting too hard to balance the two. So, I felt like I wasn't doing what the state wanted me to do and I really wasn't doing what I thought was right, which created this constant inner conflict with myself."

This seems to be a recurring issue for many teachers, not just special educators. The dilemma of not feeling that they are able to teach in the way that would best suit their students due to a singular focus on state standards for curriculum. I do not profess to have the solution to this problem, but I do think it makes a lot of sense to reevaluate these standards for students with special needs.

"I also think it's true that everybody has a right to graduate from high school and be as independent as possible. Right now, you can't do both," she added.

With that being said, Cindy acknowledged that this is not a 'black and white' issue. There is room for adjustments depending on the individual. It may be a little much to ask each state to develop personalized plans for every student— I get that. But, for someone with specific disabilities and/or cognitive impairments, I don't see the logic in saying 'all students must do X' without considering what is best for the individual. Cindy agreed and expanded on this point.

> "I'll take Will as an example—he knew so much about what was going on in the world, so he deserves to be in that Social Studies/Current Events class. In that case, I'd go and talk with the teacher and tell them 'hey look, I know he's not cognitively where your students are, but he knows a lot. And I think he could learn a lot from your classroom.' So, if somebody loves science, social studies, art, etc. I want to make sure that they are in those classes," she said.

Overall, the takeaway is that ideally, it should be a balance for these students. Cindy and I talked about the concept of an Individualized Education Plan (IEP). In my opinion, this was the most logical way to approach it. Developing an IEP involves taking a look at each person's strengths, weaknesses, where they are cognitively and socially, and then making an appropriate plan from there. I understand that IEPs are prevalent in a majority of schools in America already, but we are defeating the purpose if overarching state standards trump the personalized plan for a student with special needs. When an IEP is written appropriately, in my opinion, it will sometimes mean the child is included directly with all typical students. In other cases, it might mean that the student spends that time on something that matters more for their life in the future.

> "Could you imagine not teaching Stephen how to cross the street?" She asked, rhetorically of course. "It was the cutest thing, he took it so seriously, *and he needed that skill.* I couldn't imagine forgoing that life lesson, regardless of how small, to have him sit in a Physics class and get little out of it."

Take a moment to think about all of the little things in life that, for a typical student, are ingrained within them by the time they reach high school. This could be crossing the street, getting themselves on the bus, paying for items at the grocery store, the list goes on and on. These are learned concepts that, by going with the 'everyone has the same standards' approach, are assumed to be known by all students. This is why we are able to stop thinking about the basics for most students and focus on subjects such as Physics, Geometry, Calculus, etc. Of course, we know that is not the case for everyone and that cannot be ignored.

Cindy added on this note that when the material is too challenging, behavioral issues begin to surface. For many of her former students, she noticed that they would begin to act out significantly more if they were in a class that was too challenging. Makes sense, right? If I were in a classroom and the teacher was speaking almost entirely in a different language, it might be difficult for me to stay engaged, too.

The curriculum is just one of many components involved for a special educator to be effective. Cindy made it a point multiple times during our conversation to note the importance "bringing the parents along with her" when working with her students. With that in mind, I asked her specifically for advice she would give to parents when it comes to working with a special educator, and how to make their job easier.

> "There are so many resources out there now, but you can feel good about talking to your intervention specialist. They became a teacher out of their passion and wanting to make a difference. So, ask them to be open with you, but I'd ask parents to look at all those resources because there are so many people online sharing their story," she said.

Later on in the book, I highlight a situation in which the parent of an individual with special needs also happens to be an intervention specialist—talk about being prepared for the tasks at hand. However, this of course is not the norm. For most parents, they are essentially being thrown into the fire with no preparation on how to go about it. So, it is crucial to understand that while there may not be a specific handbook on how to approach it, it is still possible to learn from the experience of others.

Bottom line: if you are a parent of a child with special needs, you are not alone.

Cindy went on to highlight a particular family with an Instagram page called 'Finding Cooper's Voice.' Their oldest son was diagnosed with Autism and initially, the mother had the same reaction that would be completely understandable (I am paraphrasing here, as this is from Cindy's experience of watching the woman's videos). She thought things such as 'there's not much hope and what's this going to be like for the rest of our life?' Despite those fears, she took a proactive approach to helping her son, Cooper, grow.

> "That mother had high expectations of him right from the get-go. She worked with him, she worked with the teachers, and asked all of the questions that she needed to have answered. She did her due diligence as a parent and as an educator. He used to not be able to go anywhere, not even get in the car. Now at 11 years old, he goes to his brother's hockey games, he goes to the zoo, he's invited to birthday parties, etc. So, the resources are available. I would say to parents not to wait to get educated on how to support your son or daughter because there's a lot of good out there."

My advice after hearing Cindy's depiction of this mother? If you are even remotely app-savvy as a parent, head over to Instagram and give "findingcoopersvoice" a follow. She posts consistently and is truly an inspiration for anyone that has a child with special needs. I will put a list of helpful resources at the end of the book as well, but following along with empowering people like this is a great start.

REFLECTION

We talked about the "little things" that many of us understand from a young age. What are some things that come naturally to you, that you have been taking for granted?

_____
_____
_____
_____
_____
_____
_____
_____
_____
_____

FIVE

Typical Students Getting Involved

"The best and most beautiful things in the world cannot be seen or even touched, they must be felt with the heart!"
Helen Keller

IF IT WEREN'T for the positive influence of Alex Williams, my mind and heart would have never been opened up to getting involved with Cindy's program during high school. With that in mind, I wanted to get Cindy's take on what she would recommend for any typical middle or high school students that may have interest in working with these individuals.

 First of all, I wouldn't want anyone to come into a classroom unless they felt in their heart that they wanted to do it. Don't force anything that's not natural. But, my suggestion is to give it a try because what you get back from these individuals who are non-judgmental, open, happy, thankful, generous, and loving people is so rewarding. So, if you have any inkling at all, even do something

43

as simple as observing them play basketball; they are so much fun to be around."

Similar to trying out anything that is new to you, the idea of starting small with baby steps can be a great way to gauge if it is for you or not. This is why the suggestion to simply observe students with special needs for a short period of time resonated with me. The first time I went to "Chillin' Chums," I was not in charge of facilitating a group activity or a game. I was there to observe and participate where I could like most of the others in the group.

Over time, this developed into deeper relationships with some of the students, becoming a teacher aide for Cindy, and ultimately to working as a one-on-one tutor with Stephen. I feel it is important to emphasize that the process from 'let me check this out' to 'I want to commit as much time to this as I can' took well over a full year of learning and building a better understanding of how to work with the students. And as Cindy said, more often than not, if you as a middle or high school student give yourself the time and space to 'check it out,' the rewards and impact it can have on your life (and theirs) are massive.

Of course, for the individual with special needs and their loved ones, anybody willing to spend extra time with them is much appreciated. I have heard multiple times from the Hunts, Cornells, and from other connections of mine that they've seen how much I care to make time for these individuals, and the impact I am making. I cannot stress enough that I do really appreciate that, and it definitely makes me feel good to know that others notice it. However, as Cindy and I began to wrap up our conversation, she had an important message for anyone reading this book on that subject.

"People would tell me all of the time: 'Oh you're so amazing, you're a special person to do this.' But no! The students are the amazing ones! Why don't you see that?! I wish I could tell the world that. It's fun to work with them, and I am the lucky one. Don't tell us that we are amazing people and good people —they are. And if you open your door to it, you will see that, and receive the rewards yourself."

I would imagine that sentiment resonates with anyone who has worked with the special needs community. Of course it feels good to have others acknowledge an act of kindness. There is nothing wrong with complimenting someone for giving their time to this community. The point here is that the 'you're a saint' mentality can be overstated.

SENIOR YEAR: "STEPHEN AND MITCH TIME"

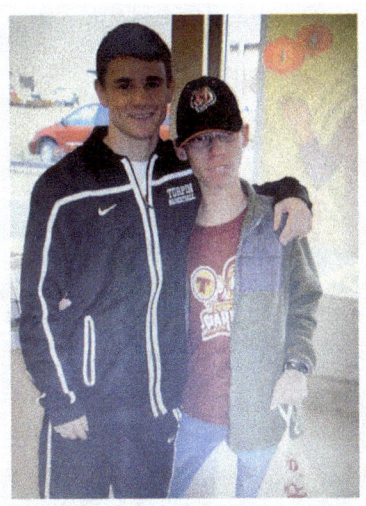

Mitch and Stephen are pictured here following a great day at the Mall.

My class schedule senior year was set up for a relatively low-key first couple hours of each day. I had one morning class, a 10-ish minute homeroom period, and then it was off to the athletic office to fulfill my 'teacher aide' duties. While I enjoyed my time working in the AD office the previous year, I was pleasantly surprised to be offered a different opportunity during that period. Cindy approached me early on in the semester about working with Stephen in art class. At the time, he was struggling to get anything done or stay focused during that period. She thought I might be able to 'work some magic' with him and turn things around.

Although I am appreciative to this day that she thought so much of me, I wasn't exactly able to make much of a change. The projects assigned in that class were too advanced for him to keep up with the group. You see, in some cases, inclusion can show up as meeting somebody where they are and working with them to make small progress. It does not mean forcing them into what a typical person is doing; it is a delicate balance. This is precisely what we decided to do for Stephen. There was no use in continuing to try the same methods over and over again for an art class that was not going to do him much good in the first place. So instead, that period became a designated one-on-one, 'Mitch and Stephen' time. It makes me smile every time I think about it.

Every morning after homeroom, I would walk downstairs to the main special education classroom and there he would be, without fail. There is not a single morning after we started these sessions that Stephen wasn't smiling and giggling at the door when I got there. When I talk about "the way someone makes you feel," this morning ritual was at the heart of it for me. It transformed my perspective on life one day at a time as I was met with the same excitement and joy every time.

This mindset shift took some time to become permanent, but I gradually became a more positive and understanding person in the process. The older one gets, the more seemingly-comical the old 'high school problems' tend to become as we reflect back on them. That is, of course, for those of us fortunate enough to grow up in safe areas with families there to provide for us. I make that disclaimer because I know for some people, the teenage years came with several legitimate, real-world struggles.

For me, however, the biggest challenges came on the basketball court or the football field. Physically-grueling days and nights of workouts, practices, being tested consistently by tough coaching—these were the biggest obstacles in my way on a daily basis. Don't get me wrong, my coaches were no joke, but my experience working with students like Stephen and Robert completely shifted how I viewed those 'challenges.' For any of these individuals, the ability to compete in a high school sport and not be left out would be a *privilege*, and one that unfortunately was not possible.

Despite the many obstacles and lack of opportunity in most areas of life, seeing Stephen's daily positive attitude was infectious.

It used to break my heart when I would think about the above concept. It still does to some extent. With that being said, it truly accentuates the extremely positive, loving-life-mentality that I have seen in so many like them. And trust me, if you would have walked down those Turpin High School stairs each morning to see that big, goofy smile waiting for you— for no reason other than excitement to spend the time with you each day—you would feel the same way.

After a couple of weeks together, Steve and I had a pretty solid routine going. The only thing he truly wanted to do? Throw the ball back and forth out in the hallway. It started with one specific day in which we were practicing some vocabulary cards. Stephen did especially well and took care of what we had down on the agenda for the day, so I asked Mrs. Gajus if we had a way to reward his hard work. About a minute later, I was the starting pitcher and Stephen my catcher.

The more seriously I took my imaginary role for the Cincinnati Reds, the harder he would laugh at me. Honestly, I don't blame him at all for being hyper-focused on wanting to do this, because it quickly became my favorite 10-20 minutes of every day.

We always had a great time with each other, but the ability to move away from mentally strenuous activity was crucial. When we could take breaks to focus on play is when it started to occur to me: this is what individuals like Stephen need. Is it important to tackle the curriculum with these students? Absolutely. I am not suggesting that we turn our high schools into playgrounds. At the same time, that aspect of "play" gets missed and undervalued considerably.

These pauses during the day in which Stephen could have fun, laugh, and throw the ball back and forth with his friend brought pure joy. To me, that matters.

I am not advocating for an overhaul of our current special education system. I also do not have the facts on how every program in America operates. This is more of a suggestion for teachers and typical students alike to make a conscious effort to bring joy to these individual's days. For teachers—if you're not already doing this, can you carve out five or ten minutes at the end of each period for some type of game to help these students enjoy their days a little bit more? Maybe it's something that fits with the topic from the day as Cindy shared earlier.

And if your current administration doesn't allow for this, well, maybe I am calling for some type of change in that case. I recently listened to a podcast entitled 'Freakonomics,' which featured American economist and Harvard professor, Roland Fryer. Fryer has years of experience studying data with an ultimate goal of improving the lives and well-being primarily of African Americans. The reason I bring this up is that one of his focus areas is improving how students are educated in America in general. According to Fryer's research, there are five core tenants that make 'good schools good'– they are as follows:

1. Spending more time in school or as he calls it, "basic physics of education."
2. Use data to drive instruction– having a real plan to make adjustments and reteach certain lessons if the results are not satisfactory.
3. Small group instruction. When tutoring kids in groups of six or fewer at least four times a week, test scores were much higher in his research.
4. Human capital: how the school selects, retains, and develops teachers, particularly taking teacher feedback seriously to inform decisions.
5. Culture of high expectations. Fryer said that many of the best schools in his study "knew that they were dealing with high poverty rates, many single-family households, etc. But, they didn't use it as an excuse not to teach."

To piggyback off of his last point, I'd submit that many of the best *special education programs* understand the challenges at hand, but don't use it as an excuse not to hold their kids to high expectations. Tasked with teaching a classroom of students with wide-ranging special needs, as in the case of Cindy

Gajus' middle-school role, her team certainly embodied this concept.

"I really believe that kids will live up or down to the level of your expectations," Fryer added.

I believe that these five tenants can improve schools in general, but specifically when it comes to students with special needs. I am not a teacher, and I do not have years of experience in this field. However, as it relates to the topic of bringing joy to a student with special needs on a daily basis while helping them to learn something at the same time, I do know one thing:

> *I did it every day, only for one hour, and only for one school year of my life. The result? A lifelong friendship and an experience I draw from constantly when dealing with any type of struggle. So take it from me— it's worth it for them, and it's worth it for you.*

Personal Growth Strategy: A Suggestion for Readers and Teachers Alike

Another strategy I would suggest for schools (and all people in general, for that matter) to implement is called the *Miracle Morning*. This is a daily routine that was coined by author, speaker, and success coach Hal Elrod. I have followed Hal's content for several years as he works to inspire others and 'elevate the consciousness of humanity, one morning at a time.'

I know that some of you may be currently giving me a collective eye-roll, but hear me out. I am not about to suggest that everyone needs to be up at 4am with a cold shower, followed by a ten-mile jaunt around the neighborhood. This morning routine is designed simply to help you work on yourself to start your day, even if you only do one or two of the six components below, which he turned into an easy-to-remember acronym: SAVERS. They are as follows:

S- Silence (*meditate, pray, etc.*)
A- Affirmations
V- Visualization
E- Exercise
R- Reading
S- Scribing (*journal, practice gratitude*)

These are the most tried-and-true personal development practices, and Hal decided to put them together into one daily ritual. Long story short, implementing it was life-changing for him; it has been for me, too. In terms of application for schools, as little as one to two minutes can be spent on each of the 'SAVERS' at the beginning of the day.

In a recent episode of his podcast, *Achieve Your Goals*, Hal shared the story of the PS 35Q Nathaniel Woodhull School in Queens, New York implementing the *Miracle Morning*. The principal of this school, Aneesha Jacko, has been leading the SAVERS over the loudspeaker for her elementary school students daily. She reported that "her school had gone from one of the worst schools in the district in terms of detentions and suspensions, to having ZERO detentions/suspension over a three month period."

This development was a major factor in over 200 schools in the state of New York adopting the routine. It is a simple, yet profound idea to have students taking time before the day begins to center themselves and develop a focus on personal growth.

A co-author of Hal's, Brianna Greenspan, has led the charge in this effort to get schools utilizing the approach. Greenspan is perfect for the role, given that she was diagnosed with Ehlers-Danlos Syndrome, a genetic connective tissue disorder that is only now becoming more widely recognized, at the age of 23. Since her diagnosis, she has been "using the power of positive affirmations and powerful mindset shifts to overcome the inherent obstacles of her condition."

With that being said, this program is something worth considering for all schools, particularly those with special education programs.

To learn more about the Miracle Morning and/or Brianna's mission, please visit **www.briannagreenspan.com**.

REFLECTION

What did you think of the "SAVERS" routine?

If you plan to implement this: What will your new morning routine consist of and when will you start applying it?

SIX

Inclusion Beyond the Classroom

"When someone makes time for you, appreciate it. And when you make time for others, do it with sincerity, because in the end, time is the most genuine way to show someone they matter."
Rebecca Baker

It was October, 2012 at the M.E. Lyons YMCA in Cincinnati, OH. The gym was completely filled with Halloween decorations. The music was bumpin' as we all danced together, and there was an incredible turnout for the event.

Students and adults from all across the township were in attendance. It was an absolute blast. This was an event that I was unable to attend throughout high school because it was a Friday night during the football season. I certainly found out what I had been missing.

It was a night filled with dancing, games, and an insane amount of candy; this was Stephen's favorite part. We went to the Cincinnati Reds game the other night (as I write this) and the main thing he wanted from the concession stand was Skittles.

For those wondering, it is not easy to find many candy options at a professional sporting event. That said, a big thank you to the folks at Great American Ballpark, because we found 'em and it was the highlight of his night. Anyway, this was not an issue at the YMCA that night. Everyone had more than enough to stay consistently hyper for three hours.

The genuine positive energy from everyone involved was palpable. The beauty of inclusion at its finest. My biggest takeaway from taking part in any event like that one is always 'I should do this more often.'

One of the most well-known organizations that does a fantastic job of creating these experiences routinely is called Best Buddies. This company is "the world's largest organization dedicated to ending the social, physical and economic isolation of the 200 million people with intellectual and developmental disabilities (IDD)." I have participated in the "Best Buddies Walk" multiple times, and specifically recall making the trip to Louisville, Kentucky to meet with Stephen and his parents for the event in 2018. As was mentioned during the Kenwood Mall story, Stephen isn't exactly much of a speed-walker, so I was interested to see how this one would go. Most importantly, though, I was excited to see the three of them.

> *"We waited to tell Stephen until the day before this—otherwise he would only talk about it leading up to the event," his mother told me.*

This is a recurring theme that makes me feel special every time. As of writing this, the Cornells recently made the two-hour drive to Indianapolis to be a part of my wedding. Whether the get-together required a two-hour car ride and culminated in a big event, or picking him up to drive five minutes up the road to Skyline, that same excitement is described.

Whether it's a week-long vacation or something as small as meeting a friend for dinner, there is value in the anticipation.

Making these minuscule efforts to spend time with individuals with special needs can create that feeling for them constantly, and that brings so much joy. The actual event? Torrential downpour of rain on that Saturday morning in Louisville and it was freezing cold, so the walk didn't end up happening. We still got time together and made the most of it. Not to mention, I think Stephen was actually happier with the outcome: no long walk, and we went to breakfast together instead. Come to think of it, I don't blame him for that mentality at all.

Memories like the one described above never fade for me. I plan to continue making an effort to spend time with special people such as Stephen and Robert throughout the rest of my life. This all started with the inspiration of Cindy Gajus.

Her program was a microcosm of how inclusion and seeing beyond disabilities could permeate our communities. The key is to continue growing awareness within each community. I hope that this book can help the cause, but it's something that can continue to grow one conversation at a time.

You, reading this, can contribute in a big way by sharing these ideas with others or modeling how to act when a situation involves an individual with special needs and/or disabilities.

People have become more aware of the negative effect the "R" word, for example, can have on those close to these communities. In my own experience, I started calling it out when I saw it. I let the people closest to me know that it just doesn't sit right with me in any context. I'm not going to freak out on someone if I hear, especially because it has been a long time since I have heard someone use it with the intention of putting down someone with special needs. With that being said, I'd still bet that a majority of my friends and family now know this about me, and try to refrain from using the word at all. As Cindy would say, it is about treating these people with the respect and dignity they deserve. To me, that includes not using that type of language behind their backs, too.

I'd like to think that I've made a big impact on Stephen, Robert, and others within the Life Skills group from high school. I hope that if you are currently a student or not a family member of someone with special needs, you can do the same. I did, however, want to make sure that there was a section dedicated to the people that make the largest impact of all. If you are a parent or sibling of an individual with special needs and/or disabilities—thank you for what you have done and continue to do for your child, brother or sister. If you are an intervention specialist or teacher that actively chose to make a career out of facilitating growth and positive experiences in the lives of such people—thank you for what you have done and continue to do for your students.

As I mentioned earlier, I was a special education major in college. Several life experiences led me down a different path for the start of my career. I found other passions, things I thoroughly enjoyed doing, and the ability to help others in the process of doing them. I found a sales company that promotes inclusivity, positivity, and helps primarily young people (18-24) to grow and find themselves at a pivotal time in their lives. That career path was incredibly rewarding for me for almost a decade, and I have since moved on to a new position, also in the business world. I share this to highlight that choosing this route instead of becoming a teacher had nothing to do with a negative outlook on the teaching profession. If anything, my experience in teacher observations and student teaching only gave me a heightened level of respect for what these people do. Do I think they should be recognized, celebrated, and even paid significantly more than they currently are? Absolutely. But, that is a discussion for a different day and I'd rather focus on the positives.

Choosing to show up on a daily basis as an intervention specialist is one of the most admirable things I can imagine doing for a career. At its core, the role is to focus on helping students with the most challenges of anyone in their age group. Of course we heard earlier from Cindy Gajus, a woman who encapsulates this servant-leadership mentality as well as anyone I've ever met, but I wanted to make sure all special education teachers and family members alike were acknowledged for their hard work, care, and sacrifices, too.

You all are 'the real MVPs,' as Kevin Durant would put it. You are the ones who have supported and taken care of these individuals during their most trying times. Times at home, for the family members anyway, when your son, daughter, brother, or sister is emotionally distraught and you aren't quite sure what to do or say to make it better. Times in the classroom for the teachers when you so desperately want your student to 'get it' and be able to move on, but they either cannot or will not on that particular day.

For someone like me, spending time with the special needs community or extending a helping hand when I was in high school is something that is applauded and commended. I appreciate that. But, for those of you that are 'just supposed to,' and take that responsibility seriously — thank you all. You are truly special people.

REFLECTION

When was the last time you were so excited about something or someone that it was all you could think or talk about?

What is something that you are looking forward currently? If your answer is "nothing," take a minute to plan something now.

_____
_____
_____
_____
_____
_____
_____
_____
_____
_____

SEVEN

Disabled 365: Making a Difference in the Community

"I honestly don't even think about the wheelchair at all. It's just an 'onto the next' mentality in everything I do."
Eric Thompson

ERIC THOMPSON IS a Cincinnati native and a graduate of Xavier University. He is currently employed at Xavier and was hired to be the head basketball coach for the Varsity Boys team at New Richmond High School in May of 2022. It was important to speak with him on this topic of inclusion because he truly embodies the concept of 'seeing beyond the disability.'

Eric was diagnosed with a form of muscular dystrophy early on in life. Up until his ninth birthday he was able to walk on his own, albeit with a noticeable limp. On June 24, 1999, that suddenly changed. He suffered a broken leg at Coney Island just outside of Cincinnati.

"Just like with anyone that breaks their leg and they're in a cast, the muscles start to atrophy," Eric explained. "So it wasn't that I couldn't walk after that, but I would use a walker as much as possible. My parents held me accountable to walking as much as I could, too."

For the next four years, he used a combination of a walker, full-length leg braces, and a manual wheelchair to get around. In December 2004, he had to undergo a serious back surgery. As he recalls, it was a challenging but ultimately great decision by his parents to have it done.

> *It's a dicey surgery. Doctors do a lot of them, but it involves the spinal cord, so there is a significant risk that I could have come out of that fully paralyzed," Eric said.*

We just finished recognizing parents of individuals with disabilities, among others, for their role in this mission of inclusion and being advocates for their children. With that being said, Eric's parents deserve a special shoutout for such a brave decision with their son. If one thing went wrong during the procedure, there could be significant ramifications, but they knew it was what he needed to be as comfortable as possible throughout the rest of his life.

"At the time I obviously wasn't tickled to death to do it," Eric joked. "But, in hindsight it was the right call. Once I had that done, I really wasn't able to walk. So we focused more on maintaining arm strength and my overall quality of life, and went from there."

Eric also went on to express his gratitude for the medical staff at Cincinnati Children's Hospital and specifically his doctor, Eric Wall.

"I saw Dr. Wall every couple months for about a year after the surgery for check-ups. I haven't seen him since 2005 about it. I haven't had to follow up with it all, never had any pain or issues–truly incredible. And now, I honestly don't even think about the wheelchair at all. It's just an 'onto the next' mentality in everything I do," he said.

Given what he has been able to accomplish despite his disabilities, it is evident that he lives that mindset on a daily basis. Here are only a few of Eric's achievements that most people probably wouldn't think possible of someone in a wheelchair:

- Getting his driver's license
- Attending college out of state and getting his degree
- Getting married and buying a house with his wife, Grace
- Becoming a manager in Xavier University's basketball program
- Earning a position as the head coach of multiple basketball teams, including the varsity job at New Richmond High School

From a professional standpoint, he is most proud of that last milestone– landing a varsity coaching role. In May of 2020, Eric was featured by Fox 19 Cincinnati in a story after earning the junior varsity job at McNicholas High School, which is his alma-mater.

"His wheelchair is not a disadvantage," McNicholas Athletic Director Drew Schmidt said during the special. "There's never been an unhappy day in his life."

During this story, Fox 19 reporter Joe Danneman called this job 'Eric's dream.' While it was a major achievement, he had his sights set on bigger things.

"I would love to be my own varsity coach one day," he said. "I came this far, why not keep going?"

Two years to the day that this story aired, that dream came true. On May 25, 2022, Eric was named the varsity head coach at New Richmond. He shared with me that this opportunity means the world to him, but it hasn't come without challenges due to his disabilities. For many people, it is tough to wrap their head around 'someone like him' in a leadership role.

> "People have said to me, 'wait, so you're in charge of the whole varsity program?' And I'm thinking, 'well, aren't *all* varsity coaches in charge of the whole program? So I think there's an initial 'wow factor' for people in situations like that. I don't think it's people trying to be jerks, it just catches them by surprise and they become tongue-twisted."

Eric has a great perspective on these situations. To me, this still begs the question, how can we progress and begin to normalize people with disabilities and/or special needs getting as many opportunities as anyone else? How can we take a page out of Cindy Gajus' book, so to speak, and collectively support these individuals in pushing through their perceived barriers? I agree with Eric that most people are not actively trying to hold someone like him back by making comments like the one above. It still doesn't help. Can we start to see beyond the disability and look at these individuals through a 'can-do' lens? If so, we will actually start to see them the way that they see themselves.

> "For me with the basketball job, I think about what happens if we start losing? Does (the wheelchair) become a focal point all of a sudden? Luckily my teams have had some success and I look for that to carry on in the future, but I never want it to be all about that," Eric said.

A challenge for Eric is the mental balance between acknowledging that his achievements are uncommon, while also working to show people that this is possible for others like him, too.

> "Balancing those two perspectives is important for me," he said. "First, it comes down to recognizing that what I'm doing is different. If I don't acknowledge that, then I'm aloof to the fact and I don't want to come across that way. I try to show people with my confidence that I deserve to be here."

He then went on to speak directly about his most recent achievement, earning the varsity head coaching position.

> "The Athletic Director at New Richmond is well-respected and he has been there awhile, so it's really nice that he would go out on a limb to hire me," he started. "I got the job over two people that were qualified and would have made sense as the choice, so it means a lot. I know he had to make some tough decisions to choose me for the position. It takes a special person to do that."

Athletic Director Doug Foote truly saw beyond the disability with his decision to hire Eric at New Richmond. As I write this, he has yet to coach in his first regular season game, so all we can do is speculate. However, if history tells us anything about this man, I would not bet against Eric Thompson.

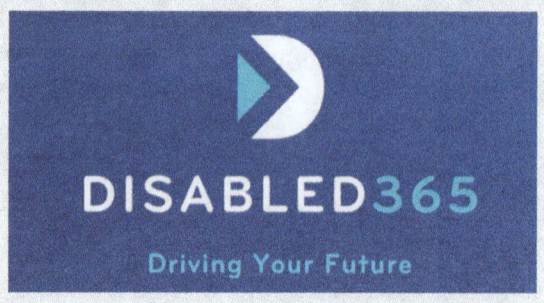

Eric is an incredibly resilient person to say the least. When asking him about what he's been able to do with his life, however, the credit is directed elsewhere. He spent most of our conversation talking about how fortunate he has been to have amazing people around him. Now, a ton of his attention is directed toward giving back to the special needs and disabled communities.

He and his wife Grace are working to make a difference in the disabled community, specifically in the area of transportation. The biggest inspiration? Their wedding night. Grace's bridesmaids bought them a ride in a wheelchair-accessible taxi, which was an extremely nice gesture. However, the cost of one ride to take them a total of 12 miles was staggering. This got the wheels turning (pun intended) for the new couple, and the idea for an impactful company was born.

> "The name of the company is 'Disabled 365.' We chose this because our mission is to help people every single day of the year, with transportation being our main focus right now. I've been extremely fortunate in having my dad and a good friend of mine who are handy when it comes to cars, so if something small happens to my van they are typically able to fix it up and help me get it back on the road. Not everybody's lucky, though. What happens if you have a job, you

drive, but your car breaks down and you have to wait two weeks? That's where we want to come in and help."

Eric went on to point out that there is a glaring need to help people with wheelchair-accessible vehicles.

"We relate to this on a daily basis. If I don't have my van, I can't go anywhere. My world is shut down essentially from an external standpoint. I've had to drive two hours to Louisville to get my van worked on because there is only one place locally, causing the wait time to be ridiculous. I was fortunate enough to be able to get my license, have a van, go to basketball practice, work, etc.," Eric added, alluding to the fact that most people with physical disabilities such as his are not able to drive or get around on their own at all. That is the issue that Eric and Grace intend to tackle with their new company.

> "I have never had a backup van, but it is a critical issue because these things break down all the time. So our business idea was to begin with a focus on non-emergency transportation; taking people to work every day, doctor's appointments, and social activities."

The need for a company like Disabled 365 is further highlighted in my conversation with Tim Hunt. He talks about his brother Robert's inability to just 'grab an Uber and meet up with friends,' which hinders his social life significantly. A service like this one would also take a massive weight off of the shoulders of the families involved.

> "Families with disabled kids need to be able to count on us," Eric continued. "And that starts with finding the right people to work for a company like this. I don't want it to be a special thing that families can

only use every now and then. The way we make the most impact on people is by being trustworthy and reliable every single day."

Eric knows that building a trustworthy and reliable company starts at the top. This is why he feels confident having his wife at the forefront.

"Grace is really the day-to-day brains behind the operation. This business is not for everybody, but our 'pie in the sky' idea for the company is being the Uber for people who cannot use it. Whether that means they are in a wheelchair, people who are disabled, or elderly people who don't necessarily trust the drivers. Our biggest challenge is hiring a staff that we can trust, are good with people with disabilities, and then from there we develop a nice training program to create trust and great relationships within the company."

Grace is perfect in this role, especially given her life experience. She does not have any physical disabilities, but chose to marry someone who does— another beautiful example of our theme here. She has seen Eric's struggles first-hand, and is motivated to make a difference within this community.

"As you know, disabilities are not a 'one size fits all' type of thing, so the ability to be flexible in that regard is critical for us," Eric said. "At the same time though, the main thing to focus on now is how are we making this safe and reliable for all users? Then, we need to make the economics work for us and for the people we are looking to help."

There are many logistical factors involved in getting the

company started, but Eric and Grace are committed to the cause.

> "If we can help a hundred people or we can help ten, we're doing alright. That's what this whole thing is about: getting to ride #1."

Eric also explained that he feels families would appreciate the familiarity of having the same two or three people picking up their son or daughter on a daily basis. It may seem like a small thing, but there is a lot of value in that type of continuity for an individual with special needs.

> "We would assign staff to geo locations, if you will. So, it may not be the same person that picks you up every time, but it could be maybe three people that are assigned to your specific area. We want it to be a trustworthy, family friendly type of thing. We would love to be that type of support system where a family could always call and get someone that they know on the phone."

The 'family feel' is something that came up multiple times as Eric described what he and Grace are looking to build. Specifically when it comes to the type of staff they want to hire, that is the focal point.

> "Like I said, the 'pie in the sky' concept is that this could become the Uber for Disabled People. But, it's a lot more intimate than that in terms of what our staff would be doing, which goes back to hiring the right people. It needs to be people that want a little flexibility, no take-home work, but most importantly, they need to want to help others. All you are doing is

helping people, making sure they're safe, and being a good person– that's it."

To illustrate one way their company could work, he gave an example using our mutual friend, Robert Hunt.

> "For someone like Robert, he could use Uber or Lyft everyday. But, those drivers are only responsible for getting him to and from, and that's where it stops," Eric said. "They are not responsible for making sure someone is safe, comfortable, etc. Getting Robert to and from work five days a week, for example, having the cost covered partially by the company he works with, partially from the family, would be a start. The ultimate objective would be that the only time Robert pays for transportation would be for social events."

Eric acknowledged that the financial aspect of making the company work has presented the most challenges. This is where he and Grace feel that it would need to be a collaborative effort to help disabled individuals, starting with companies that employ them.

> "I also think there's a huge area of opportunity from a job perspective," he continued. "I feel that places like Kroger, Fifth Third Bank, Children's Hospital, all of these places that are known to be leaders in employing individuals with disabilities, should include a small budget to help with transportation. I think those companies do a fantastic job, but it wouldn't hurt to have a little set aside to offset those needs. Otherwise, you're leaving the parent or guardian to be in charge of it, or public transportation."

He doesn't want it to be a special thing for people with disabilities to use their services. He wants it to become the norm—the obvious choice for the individual and their family.

> "We're still working out details of the type of model we want to go with, but the key is being flexible. All that families want to know is that their child is able to get from A to B safely, and we want to provide that while being affordable."

To support Disabled 365 or learn more about the company, please visit www.disabled365.com

In wrapping up our conversation, I asked Eric to speak a little more on his experience being someone who is physically disabled, but not having any of his mental faculties affected by the condition. He started by sharing that because Grace does not have any physical impairments, it has created uncomfortable interactions for them in public.

> "It comes down to being a nice person, you know? It's little things, but if Grace and I are going somewhere, people will almost always address her before they address me. For example, at the doctor's office, they'll be asking Grace, 'does he have any medication he takes?' And she's like, 'well, you can ask him!' Obviously that's really frustrating. So again, it's that ability to see people beyond the disability, to see them as the person first… that's what it comes down to for me. With my current job, for example, it's never been about the disability. It's always been 'can you do the job?' Which is how it should be."

One of Eric's oldest friends also has some physical disabilities, most notably preventing him from being able to move his arms.

> "Everyone that meets him always goes to shake his hand, but he can't lift his hand to do that. The important thing, though, is that people don't make a big deal out of it or make it uncomfortable for anybody. So again, it's being a nice person and giving people the benefit of the doubt."

Give people the benefit of the doubt. Raise your expectations of others, especially those with disabilities and/or special needs, and give them the opportunity to show you their capabilities. If we commit to these three things, as is evidenced by Eric's life achievements, the possibilities are endless.

REFLECTION

Which part of Eric's story did you find most inspiring?

_____
_____
_____
_____
_____
_____
_____
_____
_____
_____

EIGHT

Siblings: Seeing Beyond the Disability with the Hunt Family

"You have truly been my life coach and I can't tell you how much our long talks about relationships, finance, and my future mean to me."
Robert Hunt

A Conversation with Tim Hunt

WE WILL GET to my conversation with Robert's parents, Steve and Colleen Hunt, toward the end of the book. But, before we do, I had the opportunity to catch up with one of Robert's three older brothers, Tim. He has always played somewhat of a mentor role for Rob. Early in our call, he recalled the initial feelings that he and his brothers, James and Bill, experienced upon meeting their new baby sibling.

 None of us had any idea he was going to be born with Down Syndrome. Even when our parents told us, we didn't know what it was going to mean for us. I didn't feel much of a shock or that there was a new added weight to being a big brother. I was thinking 'okay I got a new younger brother,

> and he just had to have surgery on his first day of life.' That was scary because I knew at that age that surgery was something serious, but everything else seemed fine. I even remember going to the hospital and saying 'he doesn't look any different, he just looks like a baby!"

Tim was six years old when Robert was born, so it is natural that his feelings upon meeting him were highlighted with excitement and joy. He was obviously not going to have the same type of anxiety or nervousness toward the situation as his parents. Being so young, he told me that 'Down Syndrome' didn't mean anything to him at the time. The fact that he didn't feel any of those emotions, in my opinion, is a testament to Steve and Colleen's handling of the news. They described Steve being on the edge of passing out in the hospital, but clearly understood the importance of a completely different sentiment being communicated to Robert's siblings.

> "We treated him like our younger brother and it wasn't really different at first," Tim added. "There were definitely times when it was a pain in the ass," he joked. "But it taught us a much higher degree of patience and empathy than we would have received without him."

Through the early years of Robert's life, Tim recalled fondly the time they spent with each other. He was responsible in many cases for taking care of his little brother when the parents were away. This naturally led to a stronger relationship between them.

> "It was a lot, but it didn't feel like an extra burden or anything, it's just what I did. And then as he got older, started learning how to talk and developed his person-

ality, we became great friends. He is, as you know, hilarious. If he is open to you and feels like he can be himself around you, the stuff that comes out of his mouth will crack you up."

Anyone who has connected with Robert could attest to that. When he feels comfortable, his fun-loving personality is infectious. This extended beyond family life at an early age as he began involving himself with his brother's teams.

"All of the friends on my baseball team welcomed him with open arms. Immediately they saw him as a part of the team, and we became close over those early years."

This was the same thing that Steve and Colleen expressed to me about his siblings' teammates. It was also my introduction to Robert, through sports and welcoming him to our basketball team in high school. We all felt at the time that we had something special going by including Robert in everything surrounding the team.

Years later, it's amazing for me to hear that there were groups of people from an early age who were willing to do the same thing. We discussed earlier in this book some of the ways to get involved or support individuals with special needs, but to reiterate: if you're a student-athlete, please look for ways to involve these people on your team. You have no idea the impact it can have on them by being inclusive in this way, nor how much more fun you'll have by doing so.

Nobody understands this concept better than the Hunts. As they grew older, Robert continued to be a staple at their parties and team gatherings. Particularly during the time that Tim and his now-wife Tara were in their early-mid 20s

(Robert being in high school at the time), he was exposed to a fun environment nearly every weekend.

> "For a while, he'd come over on Friday nights pretty consistently," Tim recalled. "We lived in a place that used to be a nine-bedroom house, but got converted into four apartments. Three of the four units were our friends, so it really was that constant party whenever he came over. Gradually, people started moving away and the party died down, and it was tough for him to understand that."

This statement was a microcosm of what happened to Robert when leaving high school; that sense of having lost something major in terms of his social life. I shared with Tim that I, too, felt those same emotions when my high school years came to an end. Particularly as it related to sports, I was distraught for a few weeks about how much I would miss it. Those thoughts became more and more fleeting as I entered college, and ultimately I was able to move on and accept that a new chapter of life could be even better. That right there is the problem, though, because Robert and others with special needs are not as adept at processing those complex emotions.

Anyone who has spent a decent amount of time around Robert knows of his 'life of the party' attitude. At Turpin, he loved nothing more than a post-game meal with a large group at Buffalo Wild Wings, or getting the crowd going with some dance moves during a timeout in the game. These are, in my opinion, the best qualities that Rob brings to the table. Unfortunately, many of the opportunities to be that guy have evaporated post-high school.

> "We still have a good time when he's over here, but it's

definitely been different for him as we get older and it's not a party every single time he comes over."

During our conversation, we talked about the concept of losing touch naturally with friends from growing up, and the fact that going out and partying consistently is not something that continues to happen for most people. Well, trying to explain that idea to Robert is much more challenging than summing it up the way that I just did. He and others with any type of special needs will often perceive any decrease in contact with a friend in a different way. They are likely to see it through a significantly more negative lens of hurt and distrust than a typical person would. He feels left out and I can't blame him.

> "We've tried to explain this to him 100 times because we don't want him sitting around being a mope when he's upset that we aren't going out partying every night that he's here. He has come to terms with it a little bit, I think, and I do understand why he got the idea that it would always be that way," Tim added.

The impact of COVID-19 was certainly felt by every family across the country, but it had a particularly strong and negative impact on Robert. He was already losing touch with friends from high school, so to add this wrinkle almost rendered his social life 'suspended indefinitely.' Over the past couple of years, the combination of these outside factors has led to him losing a bit of his confidence in social settings. As we'll discuss later with his parents, it also resulted in him losing the desire to communicate his thoughts in general, even at home.

> "He is a riot over at our house. And then, my parents come to pick him up and he's dead quiet again. He

doesn't want to deal with having a parent or guardian around him all of the time. He wants to be 'one of the guys,' be by himself, which has been more of a development over the past couple years. I think it's natural to want to hang out more with his brothers and take advice from us versus mom and dad."

Most people can relate to this concept of being more willing to take guidance from a friend, sibling, or simply someone other than a parent that we've heard from our entire lives. This feeling is no different for Robert, but it has become more pronounced over the past couple of years. I asked Tim to shed some light on that fact, as well as to give his perspective on how he feels the changes have impacted his parents.

"It has been way more challenging since he's been out of high school. I think it's really hard on my parents because of how much harder it's been on him. What it's done for his social life, his overall attitude and demeanor has made it difficult. He just doesn't have that thing he's looking forward to every day or every week. Whether it was back in school with a basketball or football game, going to grab food with people… there was always something in the calendar when he was going to be spending good quality time with his friends. He doesn't have that now. There is no structure, and it's so tough for him to find people to do anything with. Especially when he needs a ride everywhere and might need to crash at somebody's house, it's so much more difficult than it is for you and I. For us, we can say 'sure, let me grab an Uber. I'll be there in 5 minutes,' and he doesn't live that life."

I keep coming back to the question, 'how can I show up more for Robert and other people in my life?' I think it's a great question to consistently ask ourselves. It's not like Tim sharing the above statement with me was earth-shattering information. I know how Robert must be feeling at this stage of life intuitively, yet it's still so easy to lose sight of that as I get caught up in my own day-to-day activities.

> "I don't know what it was that did it," Tim continued. "Maybe he got burnt out at work or not spending time with people and doing what he wanted to do as much as in recent years. He got into a bit of a funk, but it's getting better. He just doesn't understand why he has to drift apart from some of these people he used to spend so much time with."

There have been times in recent memory for the Hunts in which they felt like they were seeing 'the real Rob,' but the social disconnection has taken an obvious toll on him. Because of this change in his confidence level, Tim tries anything he can think of to make their time together enjoyable.

> "I know that playing rap music really loud in the car—blaring music and letting him go to town, with him acting like he knows all of the words…" he joked. "I know doing that is going to light him up every time no matter what. So that's one of those things I know will instantly make him a little bit brighter, feeling a little more like himself."

This is the concept that Susan Conroy will expand on in the next chapter: finding out somebody's 'thing' or something that gets them going and utilizing that to build the relationship.

The Best Man Speech

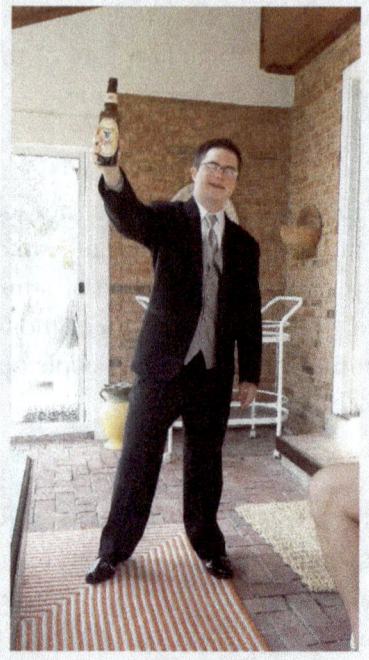

Robert gives a "cheers" to the camera as he prepares for his big speech.

When it comes to 'showing up' for someone in a big way, there are few examples better than the story of Tim's wedding party.

Whether it is somebody with special needs or not, all of us have a desire and deserve to feel appreciated and to have a 'spotlight moment' every now and then.

This is exactly what Tim provided his younger brother when giving him the honor of being his right-hand man for the big day. Given that Robert has three brothers, it was a huge deal that Tim chose him to be the Best Man. Their mother, Colleen, mentioned in our conversation that Tim has been a mentor and life coach in Robert's life. Rob was sure to acknowledge that throughout his speech. We'll get to that, but first Tim walked through the process for us from start to finish.

> "James and I were Billy's Best Men," he began when recounting the decision. "James had already planned on asking one of his best friends, and I knew that. The other part was that Rob and I have always been close, and I planned on asking him for pretty much my whole life. Because he is, you know… *he's one of my best friends. And I know that I am that for him, too.*"

The bond that these two share may have made it seem like an obvious decision for Tim, but that did not take away from the gravity of the moment when he asked.

> "I actually asked him before I proposed to Tara," he said. "I had written him this letter, so I sat him down and read it to him. At the end of it, I asked him to be my Best Man and it was pretty emotional. He was super excited and didn't know how to express what he was feeling— he was crying, laughing, trying to talk but didn't know what to say—it was a cool moment for sure."

A theme for the entire family is clearly putting in extra effort to show Robert how loved he is. It was so thoughtful of Tim to take the time to make it a handwritten letter and read it aloud to him.

> "After that, he didn't necessarily do a whole lot in terms of planning," he joked. "But, he was along for all of the fun."

I'll spare everyone any details about the ensuing Bachelor Party, but understand that Robert knows how to have a good time! Tim and I joked that he likely spent the entire year leading up to his 'Best Man duties' having fun and envisioning his big speech, at which he excelled.

> "He absolutely killed the speech. He was in his element up there and I don't know if I've heard him speak that clearly since that day," Tim said.

It was the perfect back-and-forth between sentimental and funny. The speech had me feeling all of the emotions as I watched the eight minute video clip. Rob truly spoke from the heart about his brother Tim and his new wife, Tara, but it wasn't easy to get through the speech. So, he did what I think many of us would do in this situation— he brought a beer up on stage to utilize as a bit of a bridge between particularly emotional talking points.

> "It's always been my destiny to be your Best Man," he began, between sips of his Corona light. "You have three great brothers, and I'm honored that you picked me. You could have picked any of us, and why wouldn't you? Cause, well, cause… eh, you've made the right choice."

This is one of my favorite parts of the speech, which had the entire crowd dying in laughter. It was almost as if he thought to himself for a moment, 'there are so many great things about James and Bill, where do I begin? Hmm. Never mind, good call on choosing me—onto my next point.' This sums up Rob: unpredictable, funny, and authentic at all times.

> "You have truly been my life coach and I can't tell you how much our long talks about relationships, finance,

and my future mean to me," he said, choking back tears. "I appreciate you including me whenever I ask, and it is always great to spend time with you and Tara."

He had the crowd, and myself as I watched this video, in tears at this point.

"I know there's a large group of Spartan alumni in this crowd," he continued. "Amazingly, the first night I met Tara was **THE. GREATEST. MOMENT. IN. TURPIN. HISTORY!**" He added this comment enthusiastically while beating his chest, LeBron James-style. For some background, the first night they met was when Robert scored his big basket on senior night.

The speech was heartfelt and hilarious from start to finish. Years later, it is still one of the most memorable moments as described by Tim and his parents. As he has fought through struggles with mental health the past few years, it is a moment the Hunts point to and think, 'that's the Robert we know.'

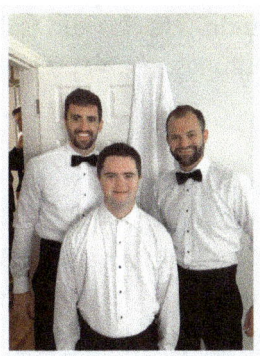

Robert's brothers, James (left), and Tim, prior to the wedding.

'Adult 101'

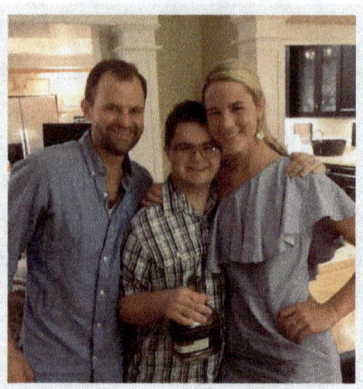

Robert's brother, Tim (left), and his wife, Tara.

Tim certainly has a focus on having a good time with Robert, especially given the struggles he has gone through in his social life. With that being said, he also understands that it can't be entirely fun and games when they are together. This is where the "Adult 101" concept comes into play. He and Tara created a list of all the little things that most adults do on a consistent basis: waking up before 10am, brushing your teeth, taking care of your own laundry, etc. The objective, of course, is to help him make these things a habit and become more independent.

> "He does it when he's at our house because we stay on him about it," Tim said. "We'll give him a hard time if he's not doing those things like brushing his teeth, going to bed at a good time, waking up earlier and showering, just taking care of himself in general."

He also added that it is not exactly easy to implement these habits when Robert spends a chunk of time at their house, and then goes back to his parents place where he may try to get away with more than he does with Tim and Tara.

> "It can be challenging to work with him when he really doesn't want to do something, so I know it's incredibly tough on my parents to keep some of the habits going."

We then discussed some of the challenges in communication and getting Robert to open up and share more of himself. I am continuing to work on making phone calls more consistent with him for the two of us to catch up, but sometimes it can be difficult to keep the conversation going or even tell if wanted me to call to begin with!

> "He has high expectations of the people around him," Tim said on that note. "One of the hardest parts, especially if you're talking over the phone, is being able to sit there and not speak on your end. You feel like, 'is he waiting for me to say something, is he going to say something?' But that patience is important. I'd also suggest if you're having a call with him, texting him ahead of time with a topic you want to talk about."

I loved this idea for anyone with a buddy or family member with special needs if you are trying to stay in touch more often, because phone calls can be a challenge. Most of the time that I talk on the phone with close friends or family members, we circle back to the same handful of topics anyway. This strategy can give some actual purpose to the call, and it gives someone (particularly with special needs) some time to prepare their thoughts on the topic.

I decided to try this out recently when scheduling a catch-up call with Robert. I let him know that my topic was going to be 'learning how to golf.' His topic? Yard work. I had no idea how this was going to go, and I thought it was funny that he chose this as a topic. As it turns out, he was 'set up' by Tim and Tara to do yard work at his parents house one day. He came home from work and much to his chagrin, his TV was missing. They then let him know that he could access the TV as soon as he pulled his weight a little more around the house, starting with mowing the lawn. Robert was not happy about this, but the Hunts are wanting to force growth in the area of independence and staying active.

Going into this call with a game plan made a noticeable difference in the quality of our conversation. He explained his frustration and I listened to the vent session. Robert felt as if his family was trying to 'make him be more like them and do these things only because it's what they usually do.' I tried to offer some perspective for him by sharing that his family only wants what is best for him long-term. This, of course, includes learning to do some of these household chores on his own.

TAKEAWAYS: PURPOSEFUL CONVERSATION

1. Have specific topics ahead of time to create more meaningful dialogue.

2. Go into it with a plan to be patient. *Let them work through all of their thoughts before interjecting.* This was a recurring theme from Tim and his parents. Practicing more patience and less interrupting gives someone like Robert a chance to actually feel heard, understood, and that his opinions matter.

I asked Tim about the possibility of Robert living on his own, given that the 'Adult 101' topic seems to be nudging him in that direction. There are, however, many factors that make this a difficult topic.

"There are times when I think he'd be really excited

about being on his own, and then there are times when I think he has the mindset of 'well, I don't mind living with mom and dad and having them drive me around, take care of dishes, laundry, etc.'"

Cindy Gajus spoke at length about an individual's natural tendency to become too comfortable living at home and having so many daily needs covered by their parents. At the same time, however, the question that comes up is this: 'does the possibility of getting too used to being taken care of beat the alternative?' The alternative for the Hunts would be constant worry over a number of issues that could occur with Rob being on his own. Tim feels, at least as it stands right now, the answer is yes— being 'too comfortable' is the better option.

> "Whether we like it or not, he currently does not do well unsupervised and taking care of himself. If he spent a month or two by himself, he would be extremely unhealthy and would not get out much. So it's a hard situation to bring up the idea of independent living without a really solid plan," he said.

The primary concern, of course, is Robert's health and safety. The other component is the actual need (or lack thereof) for the Hunts to make this move.

> "My parents feel very fortunate that they are still able to take care of him," Tim continued. "They'd rather do that than to have him on his own and worrying so much about what might happen. Just like the situation when he got robbed, people will take advantage of people with special needs. It sucks, but it's reality. So, while they can still take care of him, it's tough to make that call of getting him out there on his own."

During Steve and Colleen's section, I will detail the horrible incident he referred to above. But, the bottom line is that Tim is correct here. The unfortunate reality of our world is that there are people that will take advantage of somebody who is disabled or has certain special needs. It is nothing short of heartbreaking to think about, but a real concern for parents and loved ones of an individual with disabilities. It is my hope that anyone reading this will make the mental commitment to treat these individuals with respect, and stand up for them in a situation (God forbid) where they see something like this happening.

> "He's also not actively trying to learn how to cook or anything like that, but he likes the idea of living on his own. So, there isn't a right answer. There are so many different factors at play, and for my parents, they have to go with their gut and do what they feel is best for him."

Among those factors is the reality that this decision to live independently, if it does wind up happening for Robert, is a two-way street. It would take a full commitment and excitement level from Rob and the rest of his family to make it work, but this is not to say that it ever needs to happen.

> "My whole life I've always thought that when the time comes, Rob will come live with me," Tim said. "I don't know what the plan will be, but that's what I thought would happen and something that I'd be more than willing to do."

Tim's love for Robert and his desire to make sure he is safe, healthy, and happy truly showed up throughout our conversation. The statement above encapsulates that. Some people may think it is a given that a sibling would offer that sentiment or that they should be willing to take care of their brother or sister in the event that they have special needs, but that is certainly not the case in all families. Hearing the conviction and passion in his voice when it comes to Robert's well-being was inspiring to me, and made me honestly consider for myself: 'would I be willing to do the same?'

Susan Conroy shared the same feelings about her brother, Mark, when the topic of future living arrangements arose. While I don't know how I'd respond in that situation, these two individuals definitely have motivated me to take more action to impact people in my life with special needs.

> *"It's difficult, but as you know, it's worth it. Rob's the best, so we'll figure out whatever we need to do in his best interest."*
> Tim Hunt

REFLECTION

Who are the top 3-5 people I want to show up for in my life?

How can I go about making my efforts to do so consistent?

NINE

Siblings: Seeing Beyond Disability with Susan Conroy

"I hope this goes without saying, but I wouldn't change a thing. I've told people that when they have a little one diagnosed with Autism—I literally would not change one thing. I wouldn't want our bond to be any different than it is. Our family is lucky to have him, and we all know it."
Susan Conroy

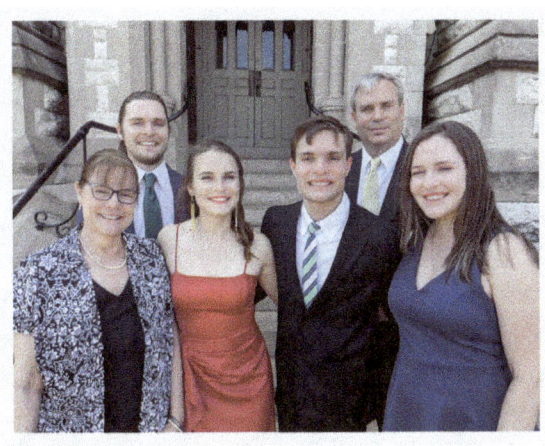

Susan Conroy (center), with her brother Mark and the rest of the Conroy family.

I sat down with my good friend Susan Conroy to talk about her experience having a younger brother, Mark, diagnosed with Autism at an early age. Their mother was a special education teacher, so she was certainly more equipped for this than your average parent. But, Susan describes her and her other siblings not necessarily thinking anything of Mark's differences early on in life.

> Early on, we were just obsessed with Mark. He was easily the favorite child for everyone in the family. My parents did a good job of easing us into understanding that things might be a little bit different. He started going to occupational and speech therapy even before his diagnosis, so (her and her siblings) got used to that being part of the routine. We couldn't drive at the time, so we'd all go together to his appointments."

This is a critical concept for any future parents out there to understand. If you learn that your child is going to have any degree of disability or extra difficulties in life, it can be a crushing blow. I'd imagine for Susan's parents, this was the case, at least to some extent. Granted, having a built-in special educator at the helm made a massive impact for their family, but choosing a positive and proactive approach to raising a child with these differences is the key here. The Conroys did such a good job of this that Susan (similar to Tim Hunt) doesn't recall any of it as earth-shattering or heartbreaking news.

> "By the time we actually got the diagnosis, it was kind of just an additional clarifying piece of information, but not really a shock to us.. He still ran the house, and he was still the favorite for everybody in our family," she added.

Transcending Labels

It was apparent even before the official Autism diagnosis that Mark was a bit behind the average child in terms of typical 'milestones' such as walking and talking. He still deals with several challenges to this day, particularly when it comes to communication with others. With that being said, he also displays some interesting quirks and impressive talents. As it relates to the quirks, Susan and her family noticed (probably because it was impossible to ignore) one of these on display early on in Mark's childhood.

He began to show that certain things would bother him that just didn't make sense. For instance, every time his mom or dad would drive him through the neighborhood, he would look to see if the neighbors had their garage doors up or down. He made a mental note of which houses usually would have the door up or down, and expected that it would be that way every time they drove past. He then would become incredibly frustrated if it was different than how he had remembered it, or in his opinion, how it was supposed to be.

It takes a high level of patience to work with an individual on an issue like this, especially when it is something that doesn't resonate with you. I don't know of any other people that become angry about the status of someone else's garage door, but this is not uncommon for an individual with Autism or other cognitive disabilities. Stephen, for example, developed a strong interest in the garbage/recycling system; it makes me smile thinking about how much he loves to talk about it.

"When is your trash day each week? Do you recycle? What color is your recycling bin?" He would often ask me, back to back, within minutes of seeing each other. There are two ways of approaching these fixations, depending, of course, on if they evoke positive or negative emotions in the individual. If it is something that they love talking and learning about, no matter how redundant, I'd suggest that it is to be embraced.

I'm sure there are other schools of thought on this, but I'd say that even if it isn't 'normal' for Stephen to be so into this topic, it is a positive thing. If it is something like Mark's inclination to become extremely upset over garage doors, however, that is where we step in and try to work past it; this is exactly what his teachers did.

> "His teachers would write him notecards that read: 'sometimes garage doors are up—I am okay. Sometimes garage doors are down—I am okay.' So I asked him about this recently, but he didn't care to talk about it. It's funny that when he was that young, he knew exactly which garage doors should be up or down and could remember all of that information."

The notecards idea is not only a practical move by the teachers, but an adorable concept to think about. And guess what? It obviously became a non-issue fairly quickly after that. Another takeaway that I had from learning this about Mark was the mental capacity necessary to remember that much information! Let me be clear— Susan described that this information caused mental breakdowns, so I am not saying that this specific fixation was a good thing for him. It is, however, another example of someone with special needs having certain abilities that may not be apparent initially.

They also will oftentimes have unique (and in many cases unexplainable) talents as a result of the way in which their brains function. Mark certainly has both of those attributes, and Susan highlighted one of his special talents as it relates to sports and recalling statistics during our conversation.

> "My mom sent me a picture of him 'doodling at school,' and he was drawing the box score for random dates in the past for Cincinnati Reds games. She went

and checked those dates for the scores, and they were all correct! He not only remembered the scores, but the hits, errors, which inning runs were scored, all of it. So I don't know where all of that stuff goes, but it's in his head somewhere."

As a huge sports nerd, this one is incredible to me. I personally pride myself on having what I feel is a wealth of knowledge specifically when it comes to football, basketball, and baseball. In certain cases, I can recall specific games, play-by-play of what happened, etc. But, the specific box score from random dates with pinpoint accuracy? No chance. That is special, and another one of those 'quirks' that certainly should be embraced. Now all we need is a winning baseball team for the poor guy :)

Now that he has moved on beyond traditional schooling, Mark is currently involved in a post-high school program entitled Pathways to Employment, which is a 'unique, comprehensive program for students with disabilities, between the ages of 18 and 22, who need a program centered on work and life skills. The program prepares students to successfully transition from school, to live and work in their community.' The objective for him is to find some type of job that works with his abilities and interests, while preparing him to ultimately live on his own. This was Mark's first introduction to the concept of a Smart Home, and he seemed somewhat excited about it. He's doing well in this program overall, but the Conroys are not necessarily in any hurry to put Mark out there on his own.

> "It's important to my parents that he has a job and is engaged in activities outside of his own bubble at home," Susan said. "I don't know if that's something we're really looking into right now. But, it doesn't mean it could never happen. He's lucky and we're

lucky that he has a support system at home. I think there's a lot of value in living in a home on his own with other people, but I also think he's engaged with a lot of things outside of home right now, so we'll see."

Upon visiting the website for Pathways to Employment to find their mission statement, I had two main takeaways:

1. I love what this company is doing for people with disabilities and the specificity with which their purpose was designed.

2. Cindy Gajus was ahead of the curve with her life skills program while students are still in high school, and it brings to attention the need for more schools to adjust their curriculums accordingly.

Susan and I both agreed on the concept that it is objectively a good thing for anybody to get the opportunity to live on their own, with one caveat: *if it truly makes sense for that individual, not to just 'check that box.'* As I talked about with Cindy, there are certain situations in which an individual is being held back to an extent or even coddled by loved ones, when they could be capable of being on their own.

Mark currently works at the Tennis Point, a local store in Cincinnati. For the Conroys, this was an important step for him— involvement within the community post-high school, as well as giving him some responsibility with having a job. After my conversation with Susan, I cannot say that this position is his dream job, though. When it comes to Mark's current dreams and desires for the future, they can only be summed up in one word: simplicity.

> "If you asked him right now what he wants to do, if he could do anything in the world, he would say that he

wants to go drive on 275, the highway in Cincinnati. He loves 275, and nobody in Cincinnati likes 275! He watches dash-cam videos of 275, and he cannot get enough of it. So things like that have definitely given me an appreciation for the simple things and looking at things a different way," Susan said.

I, too, can attest that driving on 275 in Cincinnati is not a fun time at all. However, Mark is only along for the ride and doesn't have to actually do the driving— maybe that impacts his outlook a little bit.

This is just one of many examples of Mark displaying a different perspective, something that has been a joy for the Conroy family to experience through him. That concept, in my experience, is true of all students with special needs that I have encountered; being beautifully different.

> *"Mark's been a good lesson in how everybody expresses love differently.* He pretty much exclusively communicates through inside jokes, many of which only our family would understand," she added.

One of the more hilarious examples of this occurred when Susan was running in the Flying Pig Marathon in Cincinnati. Mark came to cheer on his sister with the whole family. Throughout the race, of course, most people would cheer something standard such as "let's go, Susan!" Instead, he was yelling "thank you, Grandpa!" He directed this chant not just at Susan, but all of the runners as they passed. After the race, Susan's sister asked her why exactly Mark would be saying something that seemingly made no sense. As it turns out, he was referring to one of his favorite episodes of the children's program, Spot.

> "In this show, there is a particular scene that Mark is obsessed with in which Spot's grandpa goes up into a tree and helps to get a cat out of the tree," Susan said. "So he's yelling 'thank you Grandpa!' because in that show, they celebrate when grandpa gets the cat from the tree. So he's communicating in his own way that he loves and appreciates the people around him, but he doesn't abide by cultural and societal norms, or typical 'politeness.' He still feels normal human emotion, attachment, and bonds, it just is all in a different way."

This is crucial for anyone with interest in working with an individual with special needs. I think it is especially easy for typical students in middle or high school to simply laugh off some of these things as ridiculous and assume that the person doesn't understand the situation. Spending significant amounts of time with a person like this, however, really builds the understanding that they do know what is going on and what they are wanting to communicate in many cases, but they do it in a different way.

I have found this to be true time and time again in my interactions with Stephen. He will ask the same questions over and over again. 'When is your trash day? Where are your parents? Where are we going right now?' When I was first learning how to interact with him, I would practice extreme patience by answering those questions over and over. I can't remember when this happened exactly, but at one point I got admittedly frustrated and fired one of his questions right back at him. Here's an example from our recent time together going to the Reds game in Cincinnati.

> Stephen: Where are your parents at right now?
> Me: They're at the house!
> *Minutes later…*

Stephen: Where are your parents now?
Me: Steve, you know this. Where are they right now?
Stephen: At their house!
Me: Yes! You got it.

The key here is a different type of understanding. Through countless conversations with each other, I learned that he is retaining much more information than I initially thought. He has a few main topics that interest him, so his cognitive impairments definitely make it tough for him to generate a unique conversation quickly. It was such an amazing realization for me, though.

He just wants to talk to me as much as possible. Be patient with him and help him show how much he knows.

The same can be said for Mark and many others with special needs.

I asked Susan to elaborate on the impact that Mark has had on her family, and her answer is a recurring theme that popped up with each of my conversations: it is immeasurable.

> "He has exposed us to so many amazing people, soccer coaches, piano teachers, etc. And it's been awesome for our family to have exposure to a different community of people that we wouldn't have probably interacted with otherwise. Some of the most caring, compassionate, and kind people are in special education, so that's been great for us, too."

I agree that the type of person who is drawn to working with individuals with special needs will typically possess the character traits that Susan listed above. I'd like to add to this notion that it is also easy for one to become the type of person with a deeper level of care for others, compassion, and kindness when making the decision to build relationships with these people. So, if you're a student currently and thinking, 'I'd love to build these types of relationships, but I'm not sure how to approach it.' This is a concept that I felt was important enough to cover in each of my conversations, and I feel that Susan hit the nail on the head with her advice.

> "In a one-on-one interaction especially, anything you can do to figure out 'the thing' that the person is excited about is the key. Whether it's 275 for Mark, or taking out the trash for Stephen, anything you can do to figure that out is step one. And I don't think it takes a whole lot of digging to figure this out, either. Asking a couple questions such as 'what do you like to see outside,' or 'what games do you like to play?' Through questions like this, you can figure out what that thing is. From there, it makes it a lot more comfortable going out and doing activities with them because you have a foundation for your relationship."

She also acknowledged that this is clearly going to be a different type of foundation than you might have with other friends in your life, but I feel that is what makes it even more fun! Adults reading this: have you ever gotten sick of meeting new people with the interaction below?

'How are you? Good, how are you?' Which is usually followed up by a 'Nice to meet you. What do you do for work? Oh great, here's what I do.'

When connecting to people with special needs within your community, I promise you that there is never a dull moment within that first interaction. They are almost guaranteed to keep you on your toes. Susan elaborated on the mentality of interacting with students with special needs, which can apply to everyone reading this.

> "Going into interactions like that with the understanding that these individuals still feel emotion and have an understanding of what's going on, they just express it differently in a lot of cases. So, being open-minded about that and bringing that mentality to your interactions is the way to go."

I would add that it probably wouldn't hurt to go into *any interaction* meeting somebody new with an open mind. Sure, the differences are more pronounced in individuals with special needs, but everyone expresses emotions in unique ways.

One of the more emotional moments for the Conroy family came when Mark graduated from Loveland High School. They knew ahead of time that he was going to be specifically recognized, and Susan recalls her mother being anxious about how this process would go.

> "My mom was like, 'it'd better not be some type of Math award or something, he's not top of his class in Math and that wouldn't be fair."

I love it. *No handouts, Mrs. Conroy.*

As it turned out, the school could not have done it any better than they did. Loveland's faculty created the "Perseverance Award" just for him. This was a true testament to how much the staff and school loved him, as well as to Mark's work ethic and desire to learn and grow.

> "Mark had no idea what perseverance was, so we've been trying to work on that," Susan said. "Regardless, yeah he's different, he communicates differently, he learns differently—but, he is a hard worker, he is the sweetest kid in the entire world, and he will do anything to make the people around him happy. I

thought that award was perfectly appropriate for him."

This was a monumental moment, of course, for the Conroy family. Seeing Mark's hard work pay off and the school going out of their way to make sure he was recognized was beautiful. Susan's closing comments on what Mark has meant to her were equally as special, which is why I will open and close the chapter with it. None of the Conroys were surprised that he gave them yet another reason to be proud.

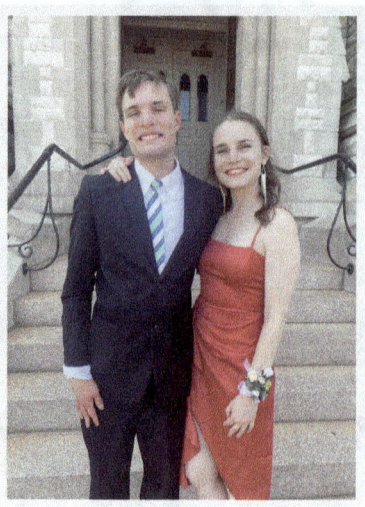

Susan and Mark pose for a shot of just the two of them.

REFLECTION

How can you apply Susan's tips for one-on-one interactions with someone with special needs?

How about with any important person in your life?

_____
_____
_____
_____
_____
_____
_____
_____
_____
_____

TEN

Parents Seeing Beyond the Disability with Steve and Colleen Hunt

"He was like a superstar right away. We had nurses come to the house to check on him when he got back from the hospital, and he was performing at a much higher level than he was supposed to in many ways. I remember the nurses saying 'wow, he can nurse, he uses a pacifier, he's got great muscle tone in his face, that is not common for most kids like him.' And I'm thinking well yeah, he's just a superstar I guess."
Colleen Hunt

ROBERT HUNT IS A SUPERSTAR, but you already knew that (see chapter one). I sat down with his parents, Steve and Colleen, to talk about challenges, moments of joy, and what it means to be a parent of someone with special needs.

 "The thought never crossed our minds," Steve said when describing the day Robert was born.

"We never really knew many people with special needs prior to having Robert. When we found out, it was a few hours after the birth, but we knew there were issues right away. We just didn't know what it was. I went down to where they take all the newborns, and I had been through this three times already with our other sons. The looks on the doctors' faces were not the same as I had experienced before. They were feverishly working on him, so I'm thinking 'what's going on?' Then, the nurse came out and said 'we're just doing some tests,' and obviously we were worried from there."

I would imagine that for many parents of a child with special needs, it is common to not know many people in this community prior to their child being diagnosed. Susan brought this up when she described the group of people her family got to meet, only because of her brother Mark. My parents expressed to me when I first started working with Chillin' Chums at Turpin that *they were never exposed to any of the students with special needs as children.* This is something that made them even more excited for me to experience something that was entirely new to myself and to them. For the Hunts and any new parents having a child diagnosed at birth, however, it is more worry and fear of the unknown than excitement.

"Colleen and I were in her room a few hours later," Steve continued. "Our pediatrician came in, which was odd because we had never even met the guy before. He came in and said 'your child has Down Syndrome,' and I literally felt a buzz go through my entire body."

"I was in bed, so I was fine, but you were ready to pass out," Colleen added.

For a new parent, so many questions immediately arise as to how to handle the situation that it can be entirely overwhelming. After being helped to a seat and calming down a little,

Steve recalls being able to gather his thoughts and seek out some advice from the nurse.

"So, that first day I asked the nurse, do you have any information that you can share with us?' And she said 'just relax, it's not time for that yet.' That was tough because I wanted to start learning about what's going on here."

It sounds like they were trying not to inundate the family with too much information and further increase the stressful nature of the situation. With that being said, I can hardly imagine how frustrating it must have been to learn this news and feel like there was nothing they could do other than to worry about the coming months. By the time they were able to bring Robert home, though, an empowered and positive mindset started to take shape.

"Our mindset quickly became 'okay, if this is the worst thing that happens, we're gonna be able to deal with it.' But then he starts becoming a baby the same way as our other kids did! And our other sons made it easier for us because they embraced him right away," Steve recalled.

The first few months were challenging for the Hunts largely due to the social implications of the diagnosis. It is one thing to come to grips with it as a couple and move forward. Essentially having to relive the news over and over in conversations with friends and family? Well, Steve remembers that being another animal entirely.

"It was obviously devastating to hear that news initially, and then you have to share that with everybody which was hard. When we found out, it rocked our world for a good 1-3 months because you're seeing people you haven't seen in awhile, I was traveling for work, and it's always brought up. It was especially challenging because most people's reaction was 'oh, I'm so sorry to hear,' but after a little while you start to get pissed about that reaction because you start bonding with him like your other children. So, it's like *'hey don't feel sorry for us.' We were treating him like we treated our other kids, and that was our approach, but it still makes you emotional thinking about it,*" Steve said.

While the initial news was unsettling, it quickly turned out to be one of the worst parts of the whole situation. The more they got to know Robert, those initial feelings began to dissipate and turn into pure joy in having another special little guy home from the hospital.

"He was like a superstar right away," Colleen told me. "We had nurses come to the house to check on him when he got back from the hospital, and he was performing at a much higher level than he was supposed to in many ways. I remember the nurses saying 'wow, he can nurse, he uses a pacifier, he's got great muscle tone in his face, that is not common for most kids like him.' And I'm thinking well yeah, he's just a superstar I guess."

I wish I could do justice to the amount of emotion behind Colleen's words above. To see the shift in her and Steve from talking about the mental struggles of first learning the diagnosis, to a new discovery that their son was going to be even more special than they could have imagined— priceless. Of course, Robert is someone that happened to display a much higher level of talent and ability than most of his peers, so that certainly contributed (and still does) to the pride his parents show when speaking of him. However, I think that this is something that all parents of an individual with special needs experience in one way or another. It can be beneficial to know for any future parents if they are dealt with a similar situation. It will likely start off as a shocking piece of news that is guaranteed to change your life. But, so much beauty will come from it when your child starts growing up and making you proud, exactly as a typically-functioning child would do.

"We then put him in an early preschool class when he was two years old with six other kids with special needs," Colleen continued. "He was a superstar in that class, too. He was the only one that could recognize his name, and we started getting all this feedback from teachers like 'you don't know how special he is.'"

The natural next step for any parent when receiving this feedback is to encourage the growth of their child. The Hunts actively looked for opportunities to immerse Robert into situations with typically functioning children, as well as those with special needs. It quickly became a balance between connecting him with other students with special needs and challenging him to get the most out of his abilities.

"That also came back to bite us a bit," Steve added. "There's part of you that says 'if he's got all of this ability, we want to help him take advantage of it.' So, we did engage him with other students with special needs, but as he got older, he was less interested in engaging and we didn't want to force that on him."

Someone please send me a link to the handbook on how to deal with that situation as a parent! On a serious note, I think that the Hunts handled Robert's level of ability as well as they possibly could (I'm not only saying that because I love this family). As I see it, here was their 'blueprint,' if you will:

- Identify his abilities and limitations
- Take advantage of the high-ability level given his diagnosis to push him and help him grow
- Immerse him into situations with both typically-functioning peers and those with special needs
- Observe carefully how he responds in each situation

- No forcing anything on him that isn't natural

The previous bullet points bear a striking resemblance to the outline that Cindy Gajus brought up for us earlier. At the forefront, this includes the concept of finding out where the student is physically, mentally, emotionally, and then promptly raising the expectations to help them grow.

Robert thrived on being social from a young age. Whether it was showing up for school or an exciting sporting event, getting around people was the key.

"He would have so much fun with the guys from the basketball team!" Colleen said. "And his brothers' friends were always coming over and playing football, basketball, etc."

"He didn't really care to participate much in sports, but *he wanted to be a part of the camaraderie of the team.* And then as he got older, he wanted to be the guy to come in and give the big speech for the team," Steve added.

Robert attended Wilson Elementary School in Cincinnati, which was different from his three brothers. They all went to Guardian Angels, a private school that did not have the resources or programs in place for someone in his situation. This was ultimately a great decision for the Hunts because the expertise was certainly there at Wilson, but it brought up the topic in our conversation of the need for all schools to make this a priority. I shared with Steve and Colleen that, in my opinion, all schools should value having programs for students with special needs. They agreed, and added that this would be so beneficial for other kids and the rest of the community, too.

> "The experience that typical kids have, such as the kids on Turpin's basketball team, and their exposure to Rob surely made their experience better. I think it makes them more caring, understanding, and when

you run into that later in life it's like 'yeah, I know how to treat this person and I know what they can bring to the table.' So it's beneficial to the rest of the community to experience kids like Rob or Stephen Cornell, and you can see that there is value in having relationships with these people," Steve said.

We're not saying we have the answers to change the structure of schools without these programs, but still feel that bringing this to the attention of people is important.

When it came to school in general, Robert absolutely loved it for similar reasons that he loved sports—being a part of something bigger than himself and connecting with others.

"He wouldn't miss a day. He would never tell you he was sick if he was. He was up, ready, and excited to get there with all of the other people," Colleen said.

This is a testament to how much joy it brings him to be around people consistently, making new friends and having face-to-face interaction with his peers. He doesn't get this as often now as he'd like, but I can tell you from experience that this is where he thrives.

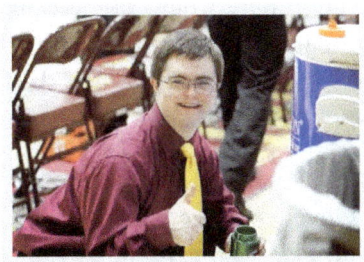

Robert gives the "thumbs up" as he dons his manager attire before a big game.

His freshman year at Turpin High School was my first real introduction to Robert. It was my senior year and he was selected to be the student manager for our basketball team. After a couple of games, Rob became somewhat of a 'Big Man on Campus.' For as little as he was able to get recognized or into the spotlight, boy did he know how to handle it when he did.

For most of our games, he led us out of the tunnel for warmups, dramatically stopping and folding his arms in a true 'tough-guy' fashion upon reaching mid-court. The first time he had the opportunity to mop up an area of the floor in front of a packed house at Klinger Court—he did. Then, he proceeded to do some type of ridiculous dance routine for another 30 seconds afterward, much to the enjoyment of the crowd.

I can vividly remember our head coach, Brad Cupito, getting all over Rob about his lack of effort pre-practice as he was going through the motions with some of his managerial duties. Some may be upset by that or find it inappropriate, but I see this as exactly what it means to 'see beyond the disability' in this context. I know the accountability, responsibility, and being pushed were all warranted and appreciated by his family. Why? Because that's what was expected of anyone who was a part of our team. Steve and Colleen recalled some of the hilarious moments involving Rob and the ultra-intense Cupito.

"Cupito told us the story, and he said something like 'effin TODAY, Rob!' The cheerleaders happened to be there, and they looked at him like, 'you can't talk to him like that, that's Robert.' It's nice that they were so sympathetic, but when we heard the story, we were happy he was treating him just as he would with any of the other guys on the team," Colleen said.

Any of his former players or assistant coaches could attest to the fact that the passion was always there with Cupito. With that being said, his main objective was helping others grow through this style of leadership. This was no different when it came to Robert.

"When we knew that Rob was going to Turpin, we ran into (Cupito) out at a restaurant one night," Steve added. "I brought up the idea of Rob being the manager and the response right away was 'absolutely,' so it was nice to have that support and willingness to bring him on," Steve said.

Cindy Gajus and I spoke at length on this concept of 'not babying' anybody and raising the standards of individuals with special needs. This is the same approach the Hunts have taken with Robert from the beginning, whether it was a situation involving a teacher, coach, boss, or another student. Steve shared that one of the best influences outside of the family on Rob's maturation was a close family friend and coach at Turpin during the high school years, Drew Schmidt.

"We were fortunate to have Drew there at Turpin because he was in school with (Rob's brother) Billy, so we knew him," Steve said. "He really was an extension of the approach we wanted to take with Rob. I told Drew from the beginning, 'you treat him the same way you'd treat your little brother if he was in the same situation, you know—if he's being a pain in the ass, tell him he's being a pain in the ass.' Letting him know when he's doing something he is not supposed to do…that surely helped him. Drew gave us a level of comfort where we knew someone would always have their eyes on him."

Another positive influence during Robert's high school years was Turpin's athletic director, Eric Fry. Fry's career trajectory aligned perfectly with Rob's schooling. He was the Physical Education teacher at Wilson Elementary, the Freshmen basketball coach at Turpin, and then ultimately Athletic

Director, so the two became very close starting in Robert's childhood.

He made sure that Robert felt included throughout his high school career, particularly when it came to the basketball team. Fry teamed up with Turpin's head coach, Ryan Krohn, to give Robert the opportunity to make that shot on his senior night. As special as it was, that moment was one of the last chances for Rob to feel the support and spotlight of the Anderson Township community.

"It is so challenging because now that he's an adult, it comes to an end," Steve said. "That whole experience we had was so positive, and it was great for the community, not just us. People are more exposed to individuals with special needs now than they were when we were kids, but there is still room for growth. For example, he still was not able to go to the same elementary school as his brothers because they did not have a program set up for it."

The further that Rob gets away from those high school years, the less connection he gets with the friends that made that time so special.

"But still, do his high school friends get how meaningful it is now?" Steve continued.

> "And I get it. You got your life and a lot going on, and you need to take care of yourself. But, there are still some people that make sure if the opportunity arises, they'll reach out—that's the hardest part, not having that. Just to include him, even get him out for a beer, it helps so much. And Robert's brothers have been so great, but we can't expect them to pick up the ball all of the time. *If you could almost set it up where someone puts it on their calendar monthly, 'reach out to Rob, reach out to whoever,' connect with that person and treat them*

like a friend. He definitely misses that, and who wouldn't?"

I think it is safe to say that I speak for any of us that were good friends with Robert during high school when I say that we do understand the importance and need for reaching out more consistently, but it is so easy to lose sight of it. The biggest key there is making it a priority and not over-exaggerating in our minds how much of an effort it actually takes to reach out and connect with our friends.

"It's always the hope as a parent that he'll have friends that will take him under their wing and check in consistently without you having to send a note to remind them," Steve said. "Hunter Sadlon (a former basketball teammate) used to have a call with him every Sunday, and he has been fantastic throughout Rob's life, but now he's moved out of town and it makes it tougher."

"I have the same situation with my mother's sister," he continued. "She's 95 years old at this point and it's on my calendar to reach out, but many times I've missed it. We used to take her out for lunch or dinner for her birthday, and we need to do it again. These are just things you need to do, and it's not specific to Rob, but with any important relationships in our lives."

Have you ever had something you were meaning to do for days, weeks, even months, and by the time you decide to take care of it, it takes you ten minutes? Or even half an hour, but you're sitting there thinking, 'why did I build this up in my head and not do it sooner?' I know I am guilty of this at times, and it is no more prevalent than when it comes to reaching out to a friend or family member to catch up with them.

As I write this section of the book, I just gave Robert a call yesterday. It was about a ten minute conversation. He gave me a few life updates even though the conversation went at a bit of a snail's pace. I'm sure he appreciated it as much as I enjoyed hearing from him. I say this to highlight the fact that it had been several months since I had last called him, and my conversation with Steve and Colleen truly reminded me that I needed to stop making excuses for myself and make this a priority.

Post-high school, Rob joined a program at Live Oaks in Cincinnati and was in a class with about a dozen other kids with disabilities. This is a great step for many kids to learn skills for life after school, but still the connection and relationships were not the same for him as they were at Turpin.

"He connected with some of those kids, but not to the extent that he did in high school. Because a lot of those kids knew him from the time they were five or six years old, so it's naturally going to be different," Steve said.

From there, he began a program with Project Search, which was essentially set up to teach individuals how to be a good employee regardless of the task at hand. According to the organization's website, the objective is that the program 'provides employability skills training and workplace internships for individuals with significant disabilities, particularly youth transitioning from high school to adult life.' So, not all that different from the mission of Pathways to Employment.

"The instructor was great," Colleen said. "She made sure that standards were clear such as 'get here on time, here's how you clock in and clock out,' and it was great in terms of showing him what life is going to be like. There is no more babying you, this is what will be expected of you in a job setting, and so on."

As grateful as the Hunts are for the many people that have

positively impacted Robert, the daunting transition to adulthood is their primary focus now.

"How do we help him to get as much out of life as he can, just like with anyone else? He's different from everyone else, and we've felt like he's kind of in a no man's land," Steve said. "He's sharp enough to realize that he can hang with (myself and our friend group), and he's done it. And he really doesn't have an interest in hanging out with his peers, even though that is getting better, but it's a constant work in progress."

One of the reasons that this is improving is Robert's involvement in group Zoom calls with five other individuals with Down Syndrome. The woman running the calls does a great job of helping them to engage with one another. Although this is a positive step, the challenge of finding his voice again is still prevalent.

The Hunt family recently moved into a new home, and early on in the process they had a disastrous flood from the dishwasher in their kitchen in the middle of the night. They woke up to the entire main floor and basement essentially ruined. I bring this up now because on one of these Zoom calls, Colleen overheard the leader of the call attempting to engage with Robert.

"I could hear her down there saying, 'Robert, are you in your basement?'" Colleen started. "And he just responded, 'yep.' It's like c'mon we just had this catastrophe! You can at least enlighten people on what happened," she said.

Steve added some insight as to why they feel this is happening.

"It's almost like he thinks nobody is interested in what he has to say. He doesn't process things as quickly, so you really have to take the time to let him get his thoughts out. This is so different from most people only wanting to get their opinion out, but you need to listen to people and give them a chance to speak. For Rob, he's not able to get out what he wants to say quick enough and in our world, people quickly move on," he said.

This is a concept we touched on with Tim, but is worth reiterating and can apply to all of us in our day-to-day interactions: willingness to listen to others without interrupting. I shared with Steve and Colleen that this is something with which I have struggled throughout my life. I'd like to think I've gotten better at it, but getting cut off in the middle of trying to say something over and over can be deflating. When you consider the emotional toll that can take on a person, you might as well multiply that by 100 when it comes to someone like Robert. It's such a simple idea, but making the conscious effort to listen to understand, not just to respond, can be especially powerful when interacting with someone with special needs.

FOOD FOR THOUGHT

Can you imagine feeling like nobody cared about what you had to say? Maybe you have felt that way in the past. How about knowing that you made somebody else feel like what they had to say wasn't important? Heartbreaking if you ask me, especially considering that I'm sure I've accidentally made Robert feel that way before. In our most recent FaceTime, I made the conscious effort to ask a question and wait as long as it took for him to say what he wanted to say. *The result? A great conversation for about 20 minutes. What a novel idea!*

"And I'm guilty of it, too!" Steve continued. "If we're all out to dinner with his brothers, Rob getting a word in edgewise is a real challenge. So, we've got a lot of work to do. I feel like he's lost confidence in that area since high school, and we're working to get that back."

Another issue on top of increasing his willingness to share is the ability to project his voice so that people can actually hear him when he does communicate. This showed up when the family took a trip recently to their lake house.

"We couldn't get him to talk, and when he did, nobody could hear him and it's just heartbreaking," Colleen added.

Steve continued on a similar note. "He's got a great sense of humor, he's a funny kid. He just doesn't share because he feels like he gets shut down a little bit. But, the other night we were at dinner and he chimed in something that was really funny. At that point it was like, 'Rob, that's you baby!' So that's what we're trying to get across to him."

My takeaway from this is that it must be a delicate balance for Steve and Colleen between encouraging him to be 'the old Rob' while not forcing it on him. It is also on the people he's speaking with to display patience and a genuine interest in understanding. As Steve sees it, too many people are quick to the have the opposite mentality:

"The minute Rob walks in the door, everyone knows that he has Down Syndrome," he said. "So already, I think unfortunately their expectations are lower and they're probably thinking, 'do I want to try to communicate with this guy? Can he even talk?'"

"It's natural for people to feel that way, but it's tough. It's a mindset of 'if I can't understand them, I'm going to shut down. I'm not going to try to engage that person because I cannot tell what they're saying right away.'"

APPLICATION

If you encounter an individual with issues communicating on a regular basis, can you practice a little more patience trying understand them in your next conversation? Clearly it makes a big difference in that person's self-esteem.

Communicating ideas effectively is a work in progress for Robert, but his ability to understand others is not a weakness, as far as I see it. At his current job, Robert works with another young man with Down Syndrome. Colleen recalled a recent story that shows his awareness of how to put another person before himself.

"It was the boss's birthday," she started. "The plan was for Robert and Ryan, who also has Down Syndrome, to take her out to lunch. Ryan asked if he could be 'Venmo'd' for it and Rob told him 'no, dude, it's her birthday so we're paying for it.' So, he gets things like that, and we're proud of that," Colleen said.

The story above ultimately brings us back to the big challenge that faces Robert and his parents: the 'no-man's land' position he is put in by having a higher understanding of social situations than most of his peers.

His heightened social IQ has impacted his expectations for dating, too. A long-term goal of Robert's is to get married one day. This presents a whole different array of challenges for him and his parents. He did have a girlfriend for a short period of time during high school, but that didn't work out as expectations did not end up meeting reality for him.

"She ended up dumping him," Colleen put it plainly. "He didn't pay enough attention to her."

As it turned out, Rob really loved the idea of having a girlfriend, but he wasn't ready for the effort it would take to make it work. The expectations concerning the type of girl he wants to date have caused some issues, too.

"Unfortunately the universe is so small in terms of girls that are his age, in this area, that have Down Syndrome, and are of his ability level, too." Steve said.

For the Hunts, this is another major reason why they are making an effort to get him involved in the community post-high school. They want to ensure that he gets out there and meets new people. Still, having those specific criteria makes it a struggle. This topic brought up a feel-good story from high school that wound up unintentionally making the situation worse.

"He asked a girl to homecoming who was so pretty," Colleen recalled. "And she said yes! It was so nice of her, so sweet, but it also adds to his frustration in that area."

This scenario hit home for me during our conversation. How many stories do we see like this every year? The student with special needs gets the beautiful prom date, scores the touchdown, makes the game-winning shot like Robert did, etc. As great as those moments are, what happens next for that person? For someone like Robert, there is a sense of 'snapping back to reality' that has had to occur each time he has experienced one of those euphoric moments.

I want to be clear that, as I alluded to in the opening chapter, anyone involved in facilitating a moment like this for someone with special needs is to be commended. It makes such a deep impact on the person and their loved ones. I also think we can be more aware of the student's emotions after the fact.

MITCH STEVENS

My hope is that people can draw from this section a greater sense of empathy for people like Robert, as well as gratitude for their own lives. So many of us (myself included) take things for granted like getting to go a school dance, try out or play for the team, etc.

REFLECTION

Is there someone in your life that "just wants to be a part of the team," but seems to get left out?

Reflect on little efforts you can make to include this person more often.

_____
_____
_____
_____
_____
_____
_____
_____
_____
_____

ELEVEN

Advice for High School Students/Treating People the Right Way

"Strong people stand up from themselves. But the strongest people stand up for others."
Unknown

WHILE I'D LIKE to think most people have compassion for individuals with special needs and/or disabilities, I understand that some do not. I asked the Hunts to offer advice to high school students on this note.

"I'd say to have their back," Steve began. "When you're in a community the size of Turpin's, there are always going to be jerks. I'm sure Rob has heard nasty things. He's never really shared that with us, but there is no question in my mind that it has happened. So, just *step up in those kinds of situations and be a leader.* I know there are plenty of kids that do that, but that would be my main piece of advice."

In 2013, an app was released by the name of 'YikYak.' The intent of the app was to give all users an equal voice and allow people to speak freely without worrying about how they would be perceived by others for doing so. When it was initially created, I was in my freshman year of college at Ohio University. I vividly remember seeing a majority of the posts on this app as negative, hateful, and flat-out giving people an opportunity to bully or put down others with no accountability.

I wasn't necessarily a big social media user at the time, but there were multiple posts I saw of students directly making fun of certain classmates of theirs with special needs. I cannot think of many things more cowardly than using an anonymous site to say something negative about another person. When you add on top of that the fact that it was directed towards members of this community? Disgusting. So, I took to Facebook along with many other angry people to speak out against YikYak. I doubt my comments did much in the grand scheme of things, but this was my attempt to be a leader. I wanted families within my circle to see my frustration for what was happening.

The app was recently re-released as of August 2021, but now the creators have made extra effort to address the issue. I want to give the people of YikYak the benefit of the doubt, particularly because I read through their entire site and can see where their intentions are as it relates to the app. However, I still don't think it's something that is realistically going to be used as a positive thing, especially when it comes to middle and high school students.

To clarify, as it stands, this is the policy from the app's website: "If someone bullies another person, uses hate speech, makes a threat, or in any way seriously violates the Community Guardrails or Terms of Service, they can be immediately banned from Yik Yak. One strike and you're out."

I love that mentality towards bullying; not giving people an opportunity to do it more than once. However, there is still no real accountability when it comes to saying something that could truly damage someone mentally. What is to stop a 13-15 year-old kid from posting one horrible thing about another student? Sure, it gets taken down immediately and that user is removed from the app. But, they never had to put their name on it in the first place! So, still not a fan.

I understand that removing this social media app from the world does not stop bullying. I am also more than a decade removed from the high school scene, so I don't have a pulse of what goes on nearly as much as I did back in 2013. I still maintain that anything that gives young people a free pass to put people down or bully others with no accountability, regardless of the overall intention, cannot be considered a positive. I share this primarily for the current middle and high school students. Just as Steve said, please step up and be a leader in these situations, whether it is at school or on social media.

In my conversation with Susan Conroy, she spoke at length about the concept of typical students realizing that those with special needs understand what is going on at a much higher level than you'd expect. Being cognizant of that fact is a crucial component to making these individuals feel safe and welcome within their communities. In the high school setting, words can do serious damage. Especially if someone is saying something hurtful towards the person with special needs, stepping in and calling it out is the way to go. Do not assume that they don't understand.

From a parent perspective, one of the things that the Hunts feel they did well was to gain an understanding of 'key players,' so to speak, that were influencing Robert consistently at school. They obviously were not able to be there all of the time monitoring every situation, but having a grasp of his core circle of influence was key. One major challenge on that same note, though, is the possibility of someone taking advantage of him as the Hunts work to allow him more independence.

> *"He's so trusting of everybody,"* Colleen said. *"I think he's starting to become more aware over the last couple of years being out in the workforce that there are actually bad people out there."*

The key players at Turpin had Robert's back and would never let anyone hurt him. Unfortunately, the same cannot always be said for the 'real world.' This showed up in a terrifying situation a couple of years ago.

> "He was taking the bus to work," Colleen continued. "And the same people were on that bus every day. We didn't know anyone on the bus, but others from Anderson Township that worked in downtown Cincinnati knew Rob pretty well. There was an incident in which a man came over to my car one day when I came to pick him up and said, 'Rob's not on the bus. He walked off with a man that none of us know. I tried to call and tell him the bus was here, but he kind of waved me off.' I was obviously freaking out."

I cannot fathom the bone-chilling experience for Colleen hearing that and being left trying desperately to reach Robert from the parking lot. I'll ease any anxiety as you read this and assure you that no physical harm was done, but some emotional scars were certainly there. Colleen broke down the full story for me.

> "All of the business people hang out in one area waiting for the bus. There are a group of other guys that hang out and listen to music with no intention of getting on the bus. Robert took a liking to a few of the guys, so he'd always hang with them while waiting for his ride home. One day, after befriending Rob over a couple of weeks, one of the men decided to make his

move. He told Robert 'I don't have any money and I need to feed my family,' so Rob pulled out his wallet. He was ready to give him anything he had, but it was only two dollars in cash. The man told him 'that's not enough, how about we go use your ATM card.'"

Even in a scary situation such as this one, the compassion and heart for others is clear when it comes to Robert. He wanted to help the man without hesitation. Little did he know that this was a special type of evil person looking for 'help.' I'd rather not spend the negative mental energy ranking 'Top 10 worst things you can do as a human being,' but we'll just say that taking advantage of someone with special needs is on there.

When it was all said and done, Robert caught the next bus home after *being coerced into withdrawing over $400 from his bank account and giving it to the man.* A heartbreaking story to say the least, but the Hunts had a great perspective on the situation in terms of the lessons it could provide their son.

> "We were obviously furious at first," Steve said of the situation. "The police told us that there was nothing they could do because he gave him the money. I was thinking 'come on man, he has Down Syndrome, he was forced to do it!'"

A different officer at least agreed to go down there and keep an eye on the area, but no real punishment followed. The Hunts quickly understood that this could have been way worse for Robert. They then redirected their attention from anger toward the man and the police to teaching him how to process what had happened.

"We had this whole big conversation with him to help him understand that this guy could have taken him anywhere," Colleen said. "He could've put him in a car, beat him up, anything. From then on, Rob was like 'wow, it is amazing that people could actually do that.' So yeah, it completely rocked his world."

Can anyone blame him there? Colleen then expanded upon how they unpacked the situation with Robert.

> "When they were crossing the street, he realized he was nervous and it didn't feel right," she said. "The guy told him 'I need this money for (pot), and don't tell anyone,' so then Rob understood he was in a bad situation and didn't know what to do."

The Hunts still feel that riding the bus was good for him. It gave him a sense of independence. Stories like this definitely validate their concerns about him living entirely on his own, though. It is a constant balance between pushing him to grow personally and keeping him safe. In speaking with the Hunts about Robert's challenges over the past couple of years, one thing was clear: going out in public with others is crucial.

> "We were snowed-in the other day and I was saying to Rob, 'here we are again with nothing to do, can't go anywhere,'" Colleen said. "And he just looked at me and said, 'welcome to my life.' That was really telling to me that getting him out there and bringing excitement back to his life is so important."

Before COVID-19 took over the nation, one of the best ways for him to 'get out there' was to join his parents at Pelican's Reef, a local restaurant and bar in Anderson Township. Remember the idea that Steve shared earlier about people immediately lowering their expectations of Robert? Well, as regulars at this restaurant, the Hunts do not experience that at all.

"We would go to Pelican's Reef on Friday nights and his thing was 'I'm sittin' at the bar,'" Colleen recalled with a laugh. "So he'd sit at the bar and we'd sit at the table with our friends, and he would talk to anybody that would sit down next to him. And the bartenders all knew him and would say things like 'hey Rob, the usual?' Which was great for him to be in that environment."

HOW CAN YOU MAKE A DIFFERENCE?

Here's what we know:

- If someone has special needs or a physical disability, it is often apparent soon after meeting them
- In many cases, people prejudge and close off communication or make assumptions about that person

What can you do if you're in that situation?

- Make an extra small effort to communicate with that person and treat them as you would anybody else. Exactly like these bartenders do for Robert at Pelican's Reef simply by saying 'hey Rob, the usual?' That small act shows him that he's being taken seriously and the person is treating him with respect.

Colleen then continued to describe Robert's outgoing nature in that type of environment.

"He actually met a woman one night from Film Cincinnati. Rob struck up a conversation with her, and then the next thing you know she was inviting him to an event the next day. Her job was to bring films from California to Cincinnati and showcase the city. She had Robert come down to join her on the set while they were filming the Netflix Ted Bundy Story with Zac Efron. He got to be in the courtroom watching the movie being made. He would be so engaging with strangers and he was able to meet people, but it's different now. I don't know if he would strike up a conversation with someone in that same way today."

The Hunts are considering getting Robert involved in some type of speech class to improve on public speaking, which is something that he has generally enjoyed doing throughout his life. The idea is to hone in on that strength and help him build more confidence in it.

"If he's got the speech written out and he practices it, he kills it," Steve said. "He introduced Dave Lapham at a golf outing in front of tons of people, did a reading at his grandmother's funeral, and even gave the Best Man speech at his brother's wedding. He did a great job with all of those."

We touched on Robert's lack of confidence in recent years being a result of losing touch with so many friends, followed by being stuck at home during quarantine. Steve and Colleen were not blaming the issues solely on forces outside of their control, though.

"We really need to help get him back in a good routine physically," Steve said. "For a while he was working out fairly consistently, and it worries me that he hasn't been doing that nearly as much. I have to be the jerk in some cases and say 'hey c'mon man, let's get up and go.' Part of that is on us, of course. We naturally give him the benefit of the doubt—as much as we try to push him, we let a lot of things slide and we can definitely improve there."

A theme throughout our conversation was that consistent coaching, direction, and tough conversations are required to help him make progress. Themes that undoubtedly show up for all parents of children with special needs. Steve recalled a glaring example of this when Robert had a girlfriend.

> "We had a discussion because he told us 'I don't know if I want to date somebody with Down Syndrome,'" Steve said. "And we had to tell him, 'well Rob, there's probably not going to be a ton of other opportunities. As much as you want to date a supermodel, that's not going to happen.' So we've tried to be as direct with him as possible, but that's a hard one."

Being direct and tackling the tougher issues head on was highlighted in Cindy's section, too. But, you never know how information like that will be received.

> "I think it's almost like he finally said 'okay, I'll give it a shot,'" Steve continued. "And it seemed like it might work for awhile, but you need to coach him all the time. So at a certain point, if he doesn't want to take the coaching, there's not a whole lot we can do."

One thing they have been able to do is lean on Robert's brothers for support in coaching him. Colleen highlighted how her and Steve particularly appreciated 'Adult 101' being introduced by Tim and Tara.

> "It's all handwritten and up on the mirror downstairs with things like 'brush your teeth in the morning' or

'when you spill a drink, get up and clean it up yourself!'"

Many of these simple things are not happening on a consistent basis. As Tim mentioned earlier, it is frustrating for Steve and Colleen when Robert makes progress away from home, but fails to follow through for them.

"At the same time, we look in the mirror at ourselves and think 'we did this.' But, there's a day of reckoning coming," Steve joked. "We probably need to have a bit of a 'come to Jesus' conversation with him to say the least."

REFLECTION

Reflect on a time in which you witnessed someone being bullied. Did you step in?

How will you be prepared to do so the next time a situation like this presents itself?

_____
_____
_____
_____
_____
_____
_____
_____
_____
_____
_____

TWELVE

Independent Living

"Not everything in life is black and white. Sometimes the best parts are gray. Just remember that not everything can fit into one your neat little boxes."
Alyssa Rose Ivy

CURRENT CHALLENGES for the Hunts have a lot to do with a lack of motivation and willingness to do some of these 'Adult 101' activities regularly. Although they acknowledged many times in our conversation that it is much easier to do some of these things for him, they know that this is further perpetuating the issues. One night recently, for example, Steve and Colleen had planned to take Rob out to dinner with them. They had a set time that they planned to leave, and made it clear to him that all he needed to do was to shave and get dressed in time to join them.

"So I went down there and he was still in the bathroom," Colleen began. "We were getting our coats upstairs, fully ready to go, so I said 'Rob, what's going on?' He was in there with shaving cream on his face, but making no progress toward actually doing it. I was at a loss. After pleading with him multiple times, I had to just shut the door and come back upstairs."

Several minutes later, he was upstairs and dressed, but still never shaved. The overall lack of a sense of urgency to get these tasks done has been a major issue for the Hunts. It is their objective to help him become self-sufficient, but it is an everyday grind for them between what is best for Robert and what is easiest at the moment. On paper, it could sound like the answer is clear: choose the harder decision now in his best interest for later, right? Not that simple. Every day working on these things, and resisting the urge to do something for him to save time is a massive challenge for anyone working with an individual with special needs.

"But then I start thinking to myself, you know what would alleviate all of this? If we would just say 'on the weekends, here is your routine. You're off of work on Fridays, so you'll get up, shower, shave, get dressed, and it's now a part of your week.' That's something that could make a difference, but it's a constant grind," Colleen said.

The situation above is something that most parents and teachers of people with special needs have experienced. A heightened level of patience can be required to help these individuals. For Robert, however, the Hunts discovered that the lack of motivation was deeper than Down Syndrome.

The COVID-19 pandemic had a lasting effect on many Americans from a mental health perspective. When you consider the toll it can take emotionally on someone like Robert, the results are heartbreaking. For a period of time, he experienced depression for the first time in his life.

"He couldn't eat, he lost a ton of weight. He went through a terrible phase that I had never seen before," Colleen said. "He kept saying 'I can't swallow, I can't swallow.' We had all kinds of tests done on his throat, but doctors continuously told us that nothing was wrong. Then you read more about it, and that can be a part of depression. You essentially mask it with certain ailments that you wouldn't otherwise have."

Thankfully, Robert is doing much better now from a personal and emotional standpoint, but there are so many things that anyone can take from this as a bit of a checkup. I like to revisit the question, *'what could I be doing to support the people in my life that mean the most?'* You can't ask yourself that question and come up with a negative answer.

This framework leads to helping more people and helping oneself. Have you ever done something nice for another person and felt bad about it afterward? Doubtful. My suggestion is to be the person that initiates the conversation or the get-together, and the Hunts feel that makes the biggest difference for Robert.

"Just to have more of a network for him," Steve said. "To have someone making a concerted effort to reach out and check in with him, go grab a beer with him when you're in town—that is the biggest thing he's missing right now."

As covered earlier, Robert currently lives at home with Steve and Colleen. Given that we were discussing some of his recent personal struggles and ability to follow the 'Adult 101' guidelines, I asked the parents to give their perspective on the idea of him moving out on his own.

"We're going through a lot of questions about living independently," Steve said. "And it's a lot of effort to find residential properties where you can have 2-4 people living together." He brought up the same 'Smart House' situation that was discussed during Cindy's conversation, as well as the unique challenges facing Robert as it relates to this.

Every family has their own take on their child living without their supervision, as has been made clear from my interviews. It is apparent that for the Hunts, it is a goal of theirs to help Robert in the process of living on his own. This is largely linked to his mental acuity as an individual with Down Syndrome. At the same time, though, his heightened social IQ does not yet equate to his ability to complete those 'everyday tasks' necessary to living effectively in a house without his parents.

"We need to have something in place if something were to happen to us, but he needs to become more independent first before that can happen," Steve said. "He can dial up LaRosas or order DoorDash, but he's not cooking anything, for example. That is obviously something that needs to change in our mind before he could be living on his own."

This is another example of the recurring battle for Steve and Colleen in their current daily life with Rob. It is not just the challenge of learning how to cook for himself, do laundry from start to finish, or take care of the dishes after a meal. It is the fact that even with tasks that he knows how to complete, it typically takes him much longer to get it done. The Hunts often find themselves tempted to take care of some of these things out of frustration. I don't blame them.

Another major factor impacting the possibility of living in a Smart Home is trying to find a group of guys with whom he would actually enjoy living.

"We like the whole concept of a Smart Home or him being able to be on his own in general," Steve said. "It's just a matter of getting him with the right mix of personalities. Rob tends to butt heads with other individuals with special needs."

I feel that this is a major area of opportunity for our communities: the ability for as many individuals with special needs to live on their own as possible. With that being said, this is one of those ideas that looks great on paper, but there are many nuances involved in actually putting it into practice.

"It really makes a difference who you have in the house," Colleen added. "Robert wants to be able to hang out with people that want to go out to the bars, get togethers, parties, etc. because he has become accustomed to that with his brothers and other friends. The other thing about the Smart Homes is that they're called that because there are monitors everywhere to keep an eye on the individuals living there. So I asked Rob about living in one, and he told me 'I don't want someone watching me all the time.' I thought hmm, I don't want someone watching me all the time, either. So, I get it," she said.

Once again, Robert's high level of functionality leaves him in somewhat of a 'no man's land' situation. He's had hundreds of experiences with typically-functioning peers, so it is natural for him to feel on the same level with those people. However, it cannot be overlooked that certain challenges prevent him from being able to live fully independently as he is right now.

"At some point in time, hopefully we can find the right mix of people and a situation that works best for him," Steve said.

Something I had not considered prior to our conversation was the financial side of the equation. Families with a child wanting to live in a Smart Home must think of the income, or lack thereof, involved in even qualifying to live in one of these places. This was surprising to me, too!

"He apparently needs to not make as much money as he makes," Colleen said. "A lot of it is state-funded with social workers coming and providing assistance, so he might make too much to where the state would say 'you can live on your own making that kind of money,' but obviously that defeats the purpose."

Robert benefits financially from being higher-functioning and able to work a job at Huntington Bank. Because of that, he cannot receive assistance from the government to accommodate his special needs at home. How do we reconcile that? Again, not saying I have all of the answers. But, I do think it is important to bring awareness to this. *Can we at least look at things on a case-by-case basis?*

"Things have come a long way," Steve added. "It used to be that someone like Robert could only have $2,000 to be eligible for Social Security and if you had any more than that, you couldn't get it. Now, there are programs where (Colleen and I) can help put money away for him with no negative impact on him."

There are clearly many components of independent living for a family like the Hunts to consider carefully before making that decision. My hope is that changes continue to be made to make it more feasible for all individuals with special needs. Maybe it could start with Cindy's idea of a program to strategically match people to roommates based on their abilities. If decisions are being made based on making the parents and/or guardians of the individual feel more comfortable allowing them to live on their own, we are making progress.

REFLECTION

What stood out to you most about the process of someone with special needs trying to live independently?

THIRTEEN

Moments That Matter Most

"The overall experience has obviously been challenging, but it has changed our lives in so many positive ways. It made his brothers more compassionate. In the grand scheme of things, when I look around at other families, I see that what we've had to deal with is a lot less difficult than what many families have had to face. I see families with children in wheelchairs or dealing with severe Cerebral Palsy, for example, and realize it could be a lot more challenging. Overall, we are so blessed to have Rob in our lives."
Steve Hunt

I'D LIKE to think I did a pretty good job in the first couple of years after high school to stay in touch with Robert and Stephen. At least a couple times per year, we would go to Chipotle and Skyline as those are the two clear best restaurants of all-time in their minds. Given that many of the football and basketball players at Turpin were still former teammates or siblings of friends, the college years saw us get together for games on multiple occasions, too.

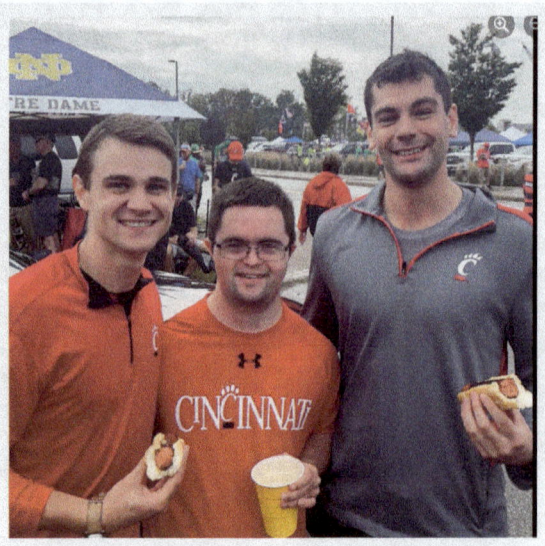

Mitch, Robert, and their good friend and teammate, Clay Johnson (right), before the Cincinnati-Notre Dame game.

However, any standard 'life has gotten busier' excuses notwithstanding, those get-togethers have lessened over the years. This is something I am committed to getting back to as I begin to approach my thirties with aspirations of having a family in the Indianapolis area. Though that may sound counterintuitive given that my two buddies are in Cincinnati, living over 100 miles from family for the past five years of my life has shown me that making the conscious decision and planning it out is all it really takes.

During 2021, I had the opportunity to bring Robert to a Reds game, as well as to attend the Cincinnati-Notre Dame football game with his family. These were two of the best days of my year, but I bring them up because it doesn't need to be some big sporting event, a wedding, party, or anything of the sort to spend time and make a difference. I can tell you that I have never seen someone taking longer to eat Skyline or Chipotle than Stephen and Rob, but those two-hour-ish lunches are some of my fondest memories with the two of them. In closing our conversation, I asked Steve and Colleen for their 'Most Memorable Moments.' Given that there are so many to choose from, it was surprising to me that they both came up with the same three immediately.

No. 1: "Boom Chicka Boom" McNicholas High School Football

"They chose a kid on the team to lead this cheer after every win," Colleen explained. "All of the fans would come back to the convent and the whole team would go up on the steps and do this big cheer. I don't remember if it was a special game or what, but they chose Rob to lead the cheer that night, and it was so special."

Rob also led the team out onto the field almost every game during his brother's senior season, and there are so many lasting memories for the Hunts surrounding that team and sports in general. McNick Football and Turpin Basketball both experienced significant success while Robert was connected to the teams. Steve thinks that there may have been 'something in the water' when he was involved :)

"He was so much a part of that football team. And an amazing thing was how much success all of the teams had. There's a part of you that thinks maybe there's something extra going on there," he said.

No. 2: "The Shot" Turpin High School Basketball

This moment was highlighted to start the book. Although nothing could compare to seeing it live, I'd recommend checking out 'Robert Hunt's Basketball Dream Realized' on YouTube. There's a good chance of tears.

No. 3: Best Man Speech

We let Tim do the honors for this one earlier. This one is particularly memorable for Steve and Colleen because it highlights what they feel is the 'real Robert.' Some of his best traits are being funny, outgoing, and truly 'the life of the party.'

No. 4: Turpin vs. McNick High School Basketball, Robert's Freshman Year

"One of the coolest things early on at Turpin was when you guys played against McNick," Steve told me. "We didn't know many people at Turpin yet, so we sat on the McNick side. We were still wondering how Robert being at a different school would go."

Needless to say, it could not have played out any better than it did.

"Guys on the McNick football team that were in the stands started chanting 'Ro-bert Hu-nt! Ro-bert Hu-nt!' And then the Turpin fans started cheering 'He's a Spartan!' And I saw Robert just light up, and I even lit up. I was starting to think, 'okay, I think this is going to work out.'"

I get goosebumps just thinking about this moment. I was on the court for it, and any current or former athlete can attest to that feeling of having a crowd cheering specifically for something that you did. Well, these moments are few and far between for an individual such as Robert (if they ever get to experience them at all). That made this one even better. Sold out crowd of close to 2,000 people, intense game on the court, yet those in attendance were focused on the special young man on the bench.

No. 5: The 21st Birthday Surprise

Steve expressed many times in our conversation the need for Robert to feel like he's 'just be one of the guys.' I feel that our basketball teams in high school took this concept to heart when it came to things like including him in team events, post-game trips to Buffalo Wild Wings or Skyline, or even something as simple as sitting with each other outside of our lockers before class. With that being said, no single event highlighted this more than Rob's twenty-first birthday party.

It was Friday, August 24 of 2019— a day that Robert had circled on his calendar for quite some time. His first Corona Light of all-time was set to be consumed. Anyway, he was less-than-thrilled with what his parents had planned for him for the big night. It was set to be a family get together, going up to Mount Lookout Tavern in Cincinnati to meet up with the usual suspects: a couple family friends, his brothers, etc.

'Greaaaaat,' I can imagine sarcastic Rob either thinking to himself or actually saying aloud to his parents. 'What a special event for my birthday. Not.'

Steve did a great job of rallying the troops and confirming that many of Robert's former teammates could make it for the surprise. I had a quick phone call with Rob leading up to the event to wish him a happy birthday and ask about his weekend plans. He wouldn't say this to me, but I know he had to be thinking: 'It's gonna be lame, why are you asking me about it if you aren't even coming?'

Maybe not, but I'd like to think I can read him fairly well at this point.

You can likely see where this is going. It was a beautiful execution of the plan from the Hunts. I drove up late that afternoon to meet up with my good buddy and former teammate, Adam, and several other of Rob's best friends were set to join us as well. It had been several months since I had last seen Robert, and I was absolutely pumped to see the look on his face. Thankfully for everyone involved, Steve captured the moment on video for us.

He met Adam and I with a look of pure joy and a huge hug, and it was one of the simplest yet most amazing moments in recent memory. The turnout for the event was incredible, too, with Robert's brothers and their friends making the effort to be there. It felt like the entire bar was there in celebration of him. I know that there were many people involved, but that in my opinion is what it looks like to show up for your child as parents. So for Steve and Colleen, kudos to you. I'm sure Robert was thinking all night about how thankful he was for you, as he slowly sipped those Coronas.

REFLECTION

Reflect on the "moments that have mattered most" in your life. Who showed up big for you?

What made these moments so special?

How can you plan to do the same for someone else in the near future?

_____
_____
_____
_____
_____
_____
_____
_____
_____
_____

FOURTEEN

From Rob's Perspective

"I appreciate how much love you have for me, and how you obviously would do anything for me. I look up to you because of the great friendships you have. I hope that will impact my friendships throughout my life."
Robert Hunt

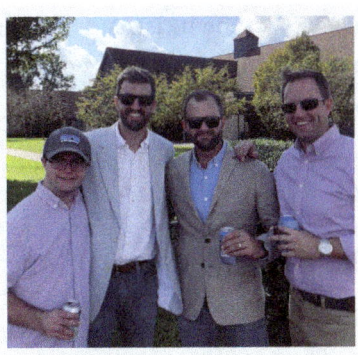

All three of Robert's brothers, James, Tim, and Bill (from left to right) pose for a group photo.

'BLESSED' seems to be the operative word when speaking to the Hunts. I sat down with Robert for my final conversation of the book, and a positive perspective on his situation was the theme throughout. Here's how the conversation went:

M: What would you want someone to know about people with Down Syndrome that they might not know?

R: "I would want to let them know that there's a lot more to us than just having Down Syndrome," he said. "I know that there is a lot more personality to me than just having Down Syndrome. *I feel that having it is a blessing.*"

Rob added the following thoughts, specifically as it relates to friends he met in high school:

"There are always people that look at it that way and treat me as normal. They don't see me as different or try to act differently because I have it."

M: What are some of the ways you feel you've been blessed to have been born with Down Syndrome?

R: "Knowing that I have so much support, whether it is family or friends. Another reason is that I would never have known any of my other friends with Down Syndrome. There are also so many social events like the independent living retreat, getting to meet really cool people like the Bengals coach Zac Taylor, etc."

M: What are your thoughts on living on your own versus with your parents?

R: "I know I'll have a lot of fun either way," he started. "I just really enjoy living with my parents. I don't have to deal with bills, first of all," he joked (kind of).

100% agree with him there, and we both got a good laugh out of it. I thought, *well yeah Rob, nobody wants to pay bills.*

Transcending Labels

R: "Another thing I enjoy is the freedom to do things I want to do, not just around the house, but also getting to hang with my own friends and my parents' friends. All of that is easier when I'm living with them."

Ultimately, it's not a goal for Robert to live on his own. He isn't completely opposed to the idea at some point, but nowhere in the near future as he sees it.

> I just know that if I lived with friends, I would have to do less of *something* to be able to make the jump to being on my own, handling bills, things like that."

M: Why does a typically-functioning person benefit from getting to know someone with special needs?

R: "You know you have friends that are going to be a good influence on you. *They have so much to give and they know how to make you feel welcome.* It also can lead to so many awesome things… If nobody on the basketball team tried to get to know me, I never would have been manager."

M: What has your family's support meant to you?

R: "For my brothers, all three of them have made a huge impact on me. It really means a lot knowing they are always there for me. To Tim, I love all the times we go see Marvel movies together. But, it's always more than just a movie to me. Just to spend time together is what matters."

To Elise, Tara, and Liz: "thank you for my nieces and nephews :)"

He then added: "I know that you will always pick me up and have my back."

Finally, for his parents…

"I appreciate how much love you have for me, and how you obviously would do anything for me. I look up to you because of the great friendships you have. I hope that will impact my friendships throughout my life."

Transcending Labels

REFLECTION

Robert shared some heartfelt thoughts to those closest to him. Who in your life needs to hear something similar from you?

FIFTEEN

The Power of Inclusion

"One person can make a difference, and everyone should try."
John F. Kennedy

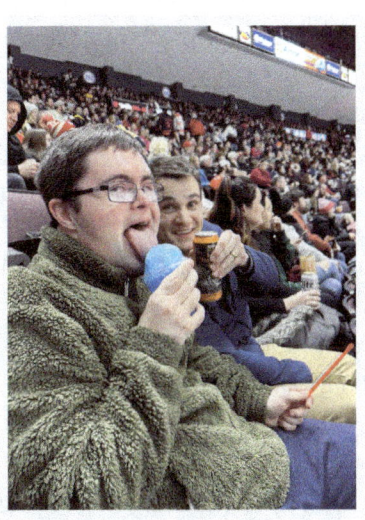

Robert and Mitch having a blast at a Cincinnati Cyclones hockey game.

THERE HAS BEEN tons of great advice throughout this book for ways that students and non-students can get involved and support the inclusion of individuals with special needs, but I'd like to wrap up with a few final thoughts from my own experience specifically for middle and high school students.

First of all, I completely understand that the teenage years can be a particularly trying time. Looking back on my middle school years especially, I can say fairly confidently that most of my actions were based on my perceived opinions of other people. From the clothes I wore, to the things I said in class, most of it was to fit in or impress people in one way or another. I bring this up because it is so easy at any stage of life, but specifically from the ages of 12-18, to be so preoccupied with yourself that you don't even see the individuals with real struggles. This was me until Alex pointed me in the direction of "Chillin' Chums" at Turpin.

As a middle or high school student, life can feel busy and stressful all of the time. On top of whatever mental acrobatics you are trying to perform to stay afloat with your peers right now, there are also several things that consistently compete with your time. You've got homework and studying (or at least I hope there is some time devoted to that), extracurricular activities like playing sports, involving yourself in clubs, potentially a part-time job, the list goes on and on. The point is that I get it, and it is not as simple in some of your situations as *"just go get involved and devote some time to people with special needs on a weekly basis, starting tomorrow!"*

Here's a simple concept that I know is worthwhile, though.

'Try it out once instead of _____, and see how you feel.' You can apply this to many areas of life when it comes to putting yourself out there and seeing what works best for you, but few things in my experience are as rewarding as the possibility of learning that giving back to the special needs community is 'for you.'

Is there an after-school club that meets once a week or even once every two weeks? Try it out once instead of going home and taking a nap, hanging out with friends, etc., and see how you feel.

Are there a couple of open seats in the lunchroom? Grab a friend, and try out introducing yourself to a couple new friends for once instead of sitting with the same group that you do every day, and see how you feel.

Do you have a study hall period during your day? Try out observing/assisting the special education teacher with their duties once instead of scrolling TikToks (I'm sure all of you guys vigorously take advantage of study hall, kidding of course) for 45 minutes, and see how you feel.

It could result in a realization that your heart's not in it, and that is okay. In my experience, however, that "try it out once and see how you feel" method as it relates to individuals with special needs has only led to positive outcomes. I cannot make any guarantees for you reading this, but I have a strong feeling that you are going to experience a sense of joy and fulfillment that makes it well worth your time. I can tell you that after my first time hanging out with the Chillin Chums group, I had one regret— not getting involved sooner.

The Special Olympics Experience

Less than a year after publishing the first edition of this book, an amazing opportunity presented itself. I was working in a sales role with an organization that is involved with a massive networking group. Throughout my time with this company, I made several meaningful connections, and it was in the back of my mind to share more about this mission. For months, however, I held back from sharing this passion in a group setting, talking myself out of it because it was not the sole purpose of any of those meetings.

The purpose is to network for my day job. My involvement with this community is separate. I'm stealing company time if I "use" these relationships for a different reason.

I don't know why we do this to ourselves. Why do we shy away from doing or saying what we desire to? Why do we hold ourselves back for fear of the worst-case scenario? There are more cliche "let your light shine," "be authentically you," or "go after your dreams" quotes hanging on the walls of our offices and homes than I care to list, yet the problem persists. It is something we "know," but often fail to apply out of irrational fear.

Finally, after much deliberation, I began to "plug" the book and why it was important to me. And surprise, surprise— everyone in those meetings was supportive and loved that I was sharing a glimpse into my personal life. It took one meeting of sharing the book and the mission for the universe to start working its magic around me. A good friend and referral partner was set to attend a breakfast hosted by Special Olympics Indiana (SOIN), and because I decided to speak up at a recent meeting, he thought to invite me. I was instantly moved and energized by the inspiring stories and people in the room that morning. I *knew* this is what I was supposed to do. I had regurgitated the lines to people around me about wanting to get more involved in the Indianapolis area, but it wasn't followed with action. This event was the push I needed. I didn't even wait until the event was over. No, instead, I walked right up to the event coordinator and asked how to get involved. She let me know that although basketball season was already well underway, I could show up the following week to volunteer and run the scoreboard for one of the games. Sold.

When I arrived at Garfield Park's Family Center the following Monday night, I was greeted with the same wave of positivity and immediate new friendships that I felt over a decade prior in Cindy Gajus' classroom. *This is where I am supposed to be.* I ran the scoreboard, enjoyed the games that night, and resolved quickly in my mind that I would continue volunteering in this capacity for the remainder of the season. A couple of the SOIN leaders who were in attendance that night had other plans.

"Is this your first time?" One of the men asked me as we were walking out of the gym. I answered in the affirmative, letting him know that it would not be my last!

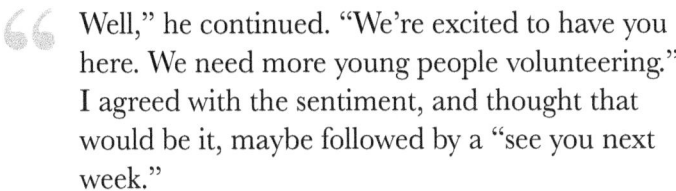 Well," he continued. "We're excited to have you here. We need more young people volunteering." I agreed with the sentiment, and thought that would be it, maybe followed by a "see you next week."

"Have you ever thought about coaching?" He asked. I beamed with excitement, as this would be the *ideal* opportunity in my mind. I love basketball and this community, and have always had it in the back of my mind that I'd like to coach one day.

"Absolutely," I said. "I'd love an opportunity to help out with coaching one of the teams."

Wow. One night of volunteering and I'm already set to coach next year.

"One of our coaches could use an assistant. How about you start next Monday?"

And so it began. On the drive home, I reflected on how a simple willingness to share my passion with others had led to this opportunity. I reflected, too, on the sad reality that this wonderful organization is *starving* for the younger generations to get involved. I snapped quickly out of the sad perspective on the situation, and came to the realization that the conversations and messages I am working to push through this book and other avenues *truly matter*.

For the next month and a half, I served as assistant coach for the Marion County South Cyclones. Working with the athletes brought so much joy, and the team even qualified for the state tournament for the first time! Flash forward to the writing of this chapter and I've completed another season with the same team, though some new players joined us this past season. The experience has been nothing but positive and rewarding. Yet another sign from God that yes, spending time in this way does make an impact, and it is exactly where I should be.

Gratitude and the Special Needs Community

How many times have you caught yourself taking something for granted in your life? If you're an average human being, you likely experience this often. I know it can be difficult to immediately shift your mind to gratitude and realize that there are far less fortunate individuals than yourself when, for example, the waitress brings your drink after a 30 minute wait or your flight gets delayed a couple of hours. I'm not suggesting that it should be easy or that I am perfect when it comes to having this type of perspective.

In my experience, though, people with special needs live in that mindset of gratitude and genuinely being present to life significantly more than a typically-functioning person. Don't we have it backwards there? That it is at the heart of why I chose to write this book. The excitement I see from Robert or Stephen when we spend time together rivals the emotion I've felt for anything I've looked forward to in my life. If I could capture that feeling and make everyone with special needs feel it every day, I would in a heartbeat. Obviously that is not possible. I can, however, choose to make a conscious effort to plan conversations and visits with those individuals, regardless of how busy my life may be. And you can, too.

For an individual like Robert, Stephen, or any one of the dozens of friends I made during my short time at Turpin, the little things are what count the most. I know it may seem cliche, but the tiny efforts made to show people like them that you love and care about them make more of a difference than you could imagine. It is tough for me not to break down into tears just thinking of it, because I am writing this as much as a reminder for myself as I am for anyone reading it. Make those little efforts to connect, especially with people in this community.

If I don't talk to my good friend Zach for three or four weeks, for example, it is fine with me because I know we're both busy and we'll catch up soon. That mindset doesn't exist for an individual with special needs.

Although this perspective is constantly offered to Rob and others like him from a place of love and understanding, that concept isn't always readily available in his mind. It feels like being abandoned by the most important people in his life if he doesn't hear from them at least every now and then.

With that being said, I hope anyone reading will take these words to heart. I hope you have used the brainstorming and reflection sections to make a game plan. My suggestion as we close out this book is to pull out something to write notes on, and brainstorm anything that comes to mind...

Who could you make an effort to talk to more? This book is about inclusion of individuals with special needs, but you don't need to limit yourself here. Anyone in your life that you wish you'd connect with more often can go on this list.

Who is the person that if you run into them out somewhere, you know you'll pick it up like you saw them yesterday, but inevitably the 'we should catch up more often' line will come up? Maybe it's a friend that moved away, a family member you only see a couple of times per year, or someone that you lost touch with because life gets busy for everybody. Call them, write them an appreciation note, shoot them a text to get something scheduled for a get-together, whatever works best for you, but do something.

Maybe writing a random thank you note to a friend or a family member is a bit out of your comfort zone, so you don't have to go that route. Consider this, though: do you know who else has written that friend or family member a random thank you note? I wouldn't be surprised if the answer is no one ever.

In a study conducted by SoulPancake, a company that was created to 'explore the ways we all seek connection, hope, truth, identity, and purpose,' the benefits of the above concept were highlighted. The study was entitled The Science of Happiness, and researchers had individuals take a test to gauge their current level of gratitude. Next, they were asked to write an appreciation letter to someone important in their life. The participants didn't know this, but after that they were asked to actually call that person and tell them what they wrote. People on the receiving end of the calls were, as you could expect, incredibly appreciative and emotional. The study showed that for those who wrote this letter of gratitude, but were unable to make the phone call for a number of reasons, they experienced an increase in happiness from two to four percent.

For those who wrote the letter and expressed their gratitude over the phone, they experienced an increase on the happiness test of up to 19 percent.

So, whether somebody on your list is like one of these amazing individuals we detailed in the book with special needs or not, this is worth your time. They will appreciate it, and you will likely experience a greater sense of happiness, too.

This is one of those concepts that we all inherently know, but often fail to put into practice.

That is the ultimate struggle in my mind: those things that are easy to do, but easier not to do.

The catch-up call with an old friend is one of those things that is extremely easy to do, yet easier not to do. Shooting Robert a text that reads 'lets go Bearcats!' when I'm watching the game? Easy to do, and also easy not to do.

So, my suggestion is to make it non-negotiable. Put it in the calendar, a reminder in your phone, whatever you need to do so that it is front-of-mind, but making a conscious effort is what matters most. Especially when it comes to any individual in your life with special needs, it is something that will make all the difference in the world.

REFLECTION

What are some ways that you could support people with special needs and/or disabilities within my school or in your community?

_____
_____
_____
_____
_____
_____
_____
_____
_____
_____
_____

Transcending Labels

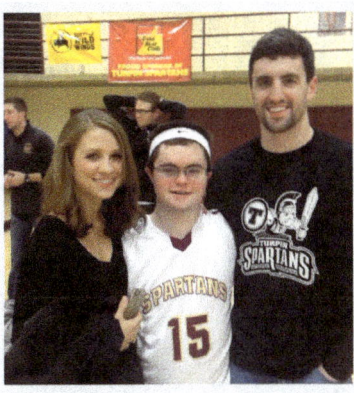

Robert gets a postgame celebratory photo with his brother, James (right), and James' wife, Liz (left)

BONUS: Blog

This section features three blogs that I wrote a couple of months following the publishing of this book.

All blogs can be found at www.mitchjstevens.com

Mental Toughness and the Special Needs Community

Do you struggle from time-to-time to keep yourself motivated? Find yourself complaining more often than celebrating the good that has happened in your days? Maybe you feel like you "can't catch a break," or you had a lofty goal, the motivation and excitement wore off, and now you've given up. By the way, feeling this way at least every now and then simply qualifies you as a human being.

Immersing yourself into the special needs and disabled communities can turn that around. How? In my experience, it is a gradual process. You get to know individuals within these communities, you learn little bits of their stories, and slowly, over time, your perspective on challenges begins to change. This has happened for me for years and years starting when I first got involved, and the beautiful thing is that the learning and growth never ends.

I had known my good friend Robert Hunt for over a decade when I sat down with his parents for the conversations that wound up in this book. I felt like I had a fairly solid understanding of what he's had to deal with from a mental and social perspective. I was wrong. Let's expand on one example from my conversation with his parents.

Rob's three older brothers are married, two of them with kids. His expectation of dating and possibly getting married have been shaped by that and what he sees on social media, in movies, etc. Here's the reality: he is not going to end up with someone that looks like any of his sisters-in-law, nor will it be a celebrity look alike. It will likely be a young lady with special needs, possibly with Down Syndrome. *That* is a hard pill to swallow.

I really want you to take a moment and consider if that were your reality. Imagine that the dating pool was shrunk down for you by **NINETY NINE** percent, there was a very specific type of person you were expected to date, and you were constantly inundated with social media promotion of women or men that *don't match up* to that expectation. So, take a moment to consider that—your husband or wife, boyfriend or girlfriend now being someone that you were so attracted to, but they were unattainable because of something you were born with.

So, as it relates to building your mental toughness in the dating arena, you could have the mindset of "man, dating is so hard, I've tried for years and can't find someone." I don't disagree with you, finding your partner for life *is so hard*, but there are two thoughts I have for you to consider.

One, is *anything* worthwhile in life easy to obtain? Absolutely not. Two, could it be worse? Could it be more challenging than your current circumstances dictate? The answer, if you are a typically-functioning person, is yes.

That second question is **so incredibly valuable** to your life. Could my current situation be more challenging than it is right now? It's a valuable question to ask yourself in terms of your overall perspective, your ability to persevere and overcome challenges, and your ability to love life exactly as it is while striving to achieve big goals at the same time. That question essentially hits the core of "is this *really* that difficult, or could it be worse, and am I being soft on myself?" It's a reality check that personally gets me out of "victim mode" and moving forward.

Example #2 is the horrible situation involving the man walking Robert to the ATM in downtown Cincinnati. That "friend" he met at the bus stop unfortunately saw this new relationship as nothing more than an easy target. He earned Robert's trust, preyed on his good heart, and completely took advantage of him.

I share and reiterate these stories not to make you feel bad about, for example, the circumstances of someone with Down Syndrome. Trust me, my friends with Down Syndrome don't spend very much time feeling sorry for themselves, so you don't need to either. There are 3 core reasons for sharing this, though.

> **1. Shift your perspective on your perceived challenges.**
> **2. Highlight what I believe is our duty as typically-functioning people to support and advocate for those who were born less fortunate than us in one way or another.**
> **3. Point out that the only way to do this is not through "awareness," but action.**

I'm guessing these concepts put your current situation specifically as it relates to dating, finding your life partner, or simply the ability to protect yourself into perspective. I'm hoping that, generally speaking with the dating example, you thought "wow, maybe I should suck it up, get out there and *try* dating because I've been feeling sorry for myself," OR "wow, I take my boyfriend/girlfriend/husband/wife for granted a little bit now that I think of it." In the second example, think about your challenges at work. For me, it comes down to job security and hopefully doing well enough to advance within my current company. The challenge of getting to and from work safely and/or avoiding a situation in which I may be taken advantage of never crossed my mind until hearing of Robert's experience. Growing your awareness of the challenges associated with the special needs and disabled communities, and shifting your perspective as it relates to your own life is step one.

The second reason is to reiterate a core belief of mine, which is my belief that as a typically-functioning person, it is my duty to support those who were born less fortunate than me in one way or another. It is my duty to use God-given abilities for good. It is my duty to be someone that, if I were ever in the vicinity of something like that story I just shared about Robert, stands up for him and literally put myself in harms way if necessary to protect against that type of evil. While all of that sounds great, the most important part is taking action.

How many times have you heard or read something from a "motivational speaker," loved the message, and proceeded to do nothing about? Everyone has been guilty of this! This leads me to reason #3 for sharing the perspective of someone with Down Syndrome struggling in the arena of love or protecting themselves. How can we help them? We can't change the situations I described, but we *can* support them emotionally. Becoming a full-time advocate for individuals with special needs and disabilities is not a path for everyone. My plea to you is to try it out once and see if it is for you. I want to spread awareness around the power of connecting with these communities, but it doesn't mean much to me if everyone *only* becomes "more aware." The only way to actually *implement* what I am talking about and make a difference is to get out there, volunteer, experience it for yourself, and truly *see* if you experience the same amazing level of fulfillment that I have.

Here are some suggestions for how you can get involved: Volunteering with Best Buddies, Special Olympics, Damar, Janus, the Village of Merici, the Down Syndrome Association, or a number of other wonderful organizations that you can find in your area. These groups are always looking for additional help! I volunteered to be a scorekeeper for Special Olympics Indiana, and was an assistant coach two weeks later!

My suggestion is to get involved by volunteering at one event. I'm confident that you'll see the joy that can come from it. People in these communities will welcome you with open arms and likely show you more love upon meeting you for the first time than any other group in your life. You leave feeling amazing. If you stay involved beyond that, genuine relationships start to build, you learn about specific challenges that Robert with Down syndrome, or Sophie with Autism, or Stephen with severe cognitive impairments have to go through. You learn about the dozens of challenges that they have to face. The thought of each individual challenge is likely more painful on its own than anything you've had to go through, and there are *dozens*. The thought of dozens of challenges more painful and difficult than anything you've had to go through is unfathomable over the course of a lifetime or a year. You learn that most, if not all, of these challenges happen EVERY. SINGLE. DAY.

So how does immersing yourself in these communities make you better? I think it's pretty clear. You're too tired? You're not feeling motivated today? The deal you were working on didn't go through? Suck it up man. Getting *dressed* this morning was tougher for many people with special needs than anything you've done in the past *month (this is my internal dialogue by the way, not calling anybody out here :))*

I draw from my experience with these individuals on a *daily basis.* From a "motivation, work ethic, overcome challenges standpoint," sure. But also from a "gratitude, love your life, perspective on what I was gifted from God" standpoint. My experience and consistent time with these communities reminds me that if my arms, legs, hands and feet are working properly, my brain is functioning at high speed, and I can see and hear clearly, then I am doing a complete disservice to the world by not doing everything in my power to fulfill my potential. To go one step further, I am doing a complete disservice to these communities if I don't use at least *some* of my time and energy to help them.

Mental toughness is a skill that allows you to do things you need to do when you don't feel like doing them, over and over again. In my opinion, it is the most important skill that any one of us can possess and continue to strengthen in our lives. My friendships with people with special needs and disabilities keep me present to that. It can do the same for you.

Should We Be Teaching This To America's Kids?

Teaching America's kids important values and concepts as early as possible matters to me; I hope it does to you, too. I am not going to get political here, but it seems to me that what we decide to add or subtract from our schools in terms of reading material is an issue that many Americans are passionate about. I'm not here to talk about your thoughts on Critical

BONUS: Blog

Race Theory, so why am I bringing this up? Well, Steve Hunt (HOF father of Rob, featured in my book) gave me the bright idea that I should begin marketing my book to schools. More specifically, he felt that the book would be particularly impactful for middle school and high school students. I love the idea, and wanted to share it here for feedback/potentially some more exposure.

Here are a couple of core concepts that the book aims to get across:

- Involving yourself and getting to know individuals with special needs will have many positive impacts on your life
- Developing empathy for others / emotional intelligence
- Individuals with special needs, just like your other peers, are able to understand and communicate with you— they just might require you to be a little more patient in learning their methods of said communication
- Bottom line: spending time with individuals in these communities is worth your time

Recurring themes that I have been hearing for over a decade are, "it makes no sense that they don't teach you that in school," or "what's the point of that being a class in our schools?" With that in mind, I feel that this would be a wonderful addition to our education system; my book would just be part of the lesson. Teachers could utilize it and ideally help students become more understanding, empathetic, and conscientiousness people in general from a young age.

As a side note, I am starting to brainstorm ideas on how I would personally structure a 2-4 week program for students with lesson plans around the book— the special education major in me couldn't help myself. More to come on that.

Two questions for you reading this:

> 1. Do you believe these would be good concepts for students to learn / have as a part of their curriculum?
> 2. How early should students be introduced to these ideas?

Please let me know via email at info@mitchjstevens.com OR direct message me on IG: @mitchjstevens.

PS— if you *do feel* that this would benefit our young people, great! If you also happen to know any connections at a school that might be able to start a conversation for me on this topic, please let me know about that via email, too.

Some Things Never Change

Some things never change— and that can be a good thing. Last week I got to spend time with my friend Stephen. Steve, Maria and I went to a bagel spot in Cincinnati.

Back in high school, I tutored him during my study hall period. Every morning after "homeroom" at roughly 8am, I made my way from the top floor of Turpin High School to the bottom. And without fail, every morning Stephen was waiting for me with a big smile. I've written at length about how this dynamic shaped my generally positive outlook on life. Not so surprisingly, last Saturday was the same. We pulled into the driveway to pick him up, and I could see him standing in the doorway with his Dad. And just like it was 2011 again (I am old), Steve was waiting with the same excitement. I figured he would be, but the confirmation in hearing him through the door was nice.

BONUS: Blog

"Oh, I think that's Mitch. I think he's probably here. Yep, I think he's coming!"

A huge smile came to my face as I approached the door. I was already excited to see him, but there's something about that same energy from him that warms my heart every time.

On the way to breakfast, we learned about the many exciting updates in Stephen's world. He still likes his job and he still stays active outside of work, currently playing baseball and participating in a Special Olympics bowling league. He still asks me the same questions about trash day, my parents, and exactly what the heck I'll be doing after I drop him off for the day. Although it was evident that some things never change, there were some new developments, too.

One of his sisters is pregnant, just like Maria! That was a fun connection for them to make. Having Maria there in general is something that has changed, too, and I'm grateful for that. While the conversations in the car and at breakfast bore a striking resemblance to those from high school, her involvement adds a beautiful wrinkle. I see him being just as excited to see her as he is me. I see her getting to know him better, and applying suggestions from my book in her interactions with him. As much as I aim to make an impact on many people through the Transcending Labels mission, the positive changes in those closest to me is what matters the most.

As I reflect on the time spent together, a few core takeaways come up for me that are at the heart of my mission. Just like the study hall period from years ago, the hour we spent together flew by. During that time, we were present with each other. During that time, I wasn't thinking about any of my challenges or what I needed to get done for the day. And most of all, when the time was up, I was left with one thought: "I'm going to make sure we do this again."

Acknowledgments

This is now the second book I have completed, so I understood the type of effort required going into it. With that being said, this one was not a 'one-man-show' by any stretch. A collection of amazing friends and family were willing to step up and support me; I cannot express how much that means to me.

To Maria: Thank you for supporting me and providing the encouragement I needed to stick with this process.

To Eric Thompson: Thank you for taking time to speak with me, share your mindset, and for continuing to inspire everyone around you. You are the epitome of perseverance and leading by example.

To Susan Conroy: Thank you for the being the first person to say yes to an 'interview' with me :) You are truly a great friend and your encouragement so early on in this process was invaluable. Mark is one lucky guy!

To Bailee Stevens, Denis McGrath, and Peggy Johnson: Thank you for your willingness to read my initial drafts and provide feedback. That part of the process is so important and helped me overcome the natural 'imposter syndrome' involved in putting out a book.

To Cindy Gajus: Thank you for inspiring me to give my energy to this community. You are the queen of downplaying any of your own achievements or contributions to your students, but everyone who knows you would speak just as highly of you as I did in this book. I appreciate you.

To Steve, Colleen, Robert, and Tim Hunt: thank you so much for giving me hours of your time, sharing your experience, and being wonderful friends over the past 10+ (wow) years. Your entire family has a special place in my heart.

To Marya Patrice Sherron: thank you for pouring time and effort into making this second edition significantly better than the first. Thank you for challenging me, and for making this accessible to more people.

Last but not least, a special thank you to the following individuals for being a part of my "launch team." I appreciate each of you for your support of this book:

Maria Stevens

Lindsay Stevens

Bailee Stevens

Kelsey Fox

Liz Johns

Zach McCormick

Katie Sedacca

Resources

Disabled 365

- www.disabled365.com

Miracle Morning/Achieve Your Goals Podcast

- https://halelrod.com/

- www.briannagreenspan.com

Freakonomics Podcast

- https://freakonomics.com/podcasts/

  ○ Episode 514

Soul Pancake: Experiment in Gratitude, The Science of Happiness

- YouTube

Pathways for Employment

- https://www.hcesc.org/pathways-to-employment/

Project Search

https://www.cincinnatichildrens.org/careers/diverse-workforce/project-search

Best Buddies Organization Site

- www.bestbuddies.org